NON-SURGICAL TREATMENT

OF DISEASES OF THE

GLANDS AND BONES

WITH A CHAPTER ON

SCROFULA

NON-SURGICAL TREATMENT

OF DISEASES OF THE

GLANDS AND BONES

WITH A CHAPTER ON

SCROFULA

By

JOHN H. CLARKE, M.D.

GYAN

Published by

Gyan Publishing House
5, Ansari Road
Daryaganj, New Delhi-110002
Phone: 011-47034999, 9811692060
E-mail: books@gyanbooks.com

Distribution Network
gyanbooks.com
India, USA, Canada, UK, Australia, France

ISBN : 978-81-212-6691-8 (PB)
First Published, 1894

2nd Impression 2022

Printed at: Gyan Press, Delhi.

Non-surgical Treatment of Diseases of the Glands and Bones: With a Chapter on Scrofula
Author: JOHN H. CLARKE

NON-SURGICAL TREATMENT

OF DISEASES OF THE

Glands and Bones;

WITH A CHAPTER ON

SCROFULA.

BY

JOHN H. CLARKE, M.D.,

PHYSICIAN TO THE LONDON HOMŒOPATHIC HOSPITAL; EDITOR OF THE "HOMŒOPATHIC WORLD," ETC., ETC.

1894.

CONTENTS.

PAGE

PREFACE, ... vii

CHAPTER I.—MY FIRST LESSON—

Case I.—Abscess in Armpit Dispersed without Operation, ... 1

CHAPTER II.—ANATOMY AND PHYSIOLOGY OF THE GLANDS, ... 5

CHAPTER III.—SURGICAL INTERFERENCE—

Case II.—Tubercular Meningitis and Death following Removal of Strumous Glands of the Neck, ... 17

Case III.—Tubercular Disease of Nasal Bones and Valvular Disease of the Heart following Removal of Glands of the Neck, ... 22

CHAPTER IV.—STRUMA OR SCROFULA—

Case IV.—Chronically Enlarged Gland in Neck Reduced by Medicine, . . 37

Case V.—Gland Abscess in Neck. Absorbed without Discharging, . . 39

Case VI.—Suppurating Gland after Diphtheria in Emaciated Child. Spontaneous Opening. Insignificant Scar, . 40

PAGE

Case VII.—Enlarged Gland following Internal Throat Affection simulating New Growth. Threatened Suffocation. Suppuration Averted by Treatment. Cure without Operation, . . . 42

Case VIII.—Enlarged Suppurating Gland allowed to open spontaneously. Insignificant Scar, ... 52

Case IX.—Enlarged Gland after Chickenpox. Suppuration imminent, but Averted, ... 54

Case X. — Post-Scarlatinal Scrofulous Glands of Three Years' Duration, . 56

Case XI.—Enlarged Glands, with Eruption on the Skin, ... 58

Case XII.—Abscess of Neck and Inflamed Glands. Action of Aconite, . . 58

CHAPTER V.—SOME CASES OF INVETERATE SCROFULA RESEMBLING "HODGKIN'S DISEASE," OR LYMPHADENOMA—

Case XIII.—Disfiguring Enlargement of Glands of Neck with very little tendency to Suppuration. Consecutive Inflammation of the Eyes. Frequent Colds. Constitutional Cure, . . 63

PAGE

Case XIV.—Chronically Enlarged and Suppurating Glands. Constitutional Cure, ... 72

Case XV.—Enlarged Glands of Neck. Inveterate Case, ... 81

Case XVI.—Inveterate Case of Scrofulous Glands. Inflammation of the Eyes. Action of Koch's *Tuberculin* and *Bacillin*, ... 85

CHAPTER VI. — NON-SCROFULOUS INFLAMMATION OF GLANDS OF THE ARMPIT. MISCELLANEOUS CASES—

Case XVII.—Inflamed Gland in Axilla from Injured Finger. Suppuration Averted, ... 95

Case XVIII.—Inflamed Glands in both Axillæ, ... 96

Case XIX.—Inflamed Glands in both Axillæ from Blood-Poisoning. Suppuration Averted. Constitutional Cure, 98

Case XX.—Inflamed Glands in Axillæ on Site of former Abscesses. Suppuration Averted, ... 104

Case XXI.—Acute Inflammation of Glands following Whooping-cough. Action of *Lachesis*, ... 110

PAGE

Case XXII.—Acute Inflammation of Glands. *Baryta carb.*, . . . 111

Case XXIII.—Abscess in Groin of Seven Months' Duration. Cured in a Fortnight with *Silica*. Operation Averted, 113

PART II.—DISEASES OF THE BONES.

Case XXIV.—Necrosis of Small Portion of Lower Jaw: Separation of Dead Bone without Operation, . . . 127

Case XXV.—Scrofulous Disease of Bones of Face, Hand, and Back. Prolonged Medical Treatment. Constitutional Cure, ... 129

Case XXVI.—Commencing Pott's Disease of the Spine. Cure by Medicines only, 138

Case XXVII.—Caries of the Spine with Paralytic Symptoms in an Adult. Arrest of Disease and Consolidation of the Spine under Medicines alone in Three Months, ... 141

Case XXVIII.—Affection of Right Knee. Suspected Incipient Tuberculosis. Cure with *Bacillin*, ... 156

APPENDIX, ... 159

PREFACE.

SURGERY is to a large extent a mechanical art. Of late years surgeons have become so accomplished that there is hardly any region of the body that is sacred from the inroads of their knives, and scarcely any disease in which they cannot find a pretext for operating. In the meantime much excuse is afforded them by the backwardness of the physician's department. Medicine proper, in the old school, as distinguished from surgery—thanks to its stupidity in refusing to learn from Hahnemann—though it has ceased to do all the evil it was wont to do of old, has learned little or nothing in the way of cure. The surgeon, on the other hand, can do something that leaves a mark. He can mend a broken limb, cut out tumours, and generally "clean up" and "straighten out" a patient. Of course he cannot cure him of any constitutional taint; but patients, as a rule, are short-sighted, and when after a decent interval their disease returns, possibly in some other form, they don't see that it is due to the inherent defect of surgery, but they start off again for the surgeon to be "cleaned up" once more.

Among the many cleaning-up operations of modern surgery, there is nothing so popular just now as the cutting out of glands of the neck when they threaten to suppurate, in order to prevent them leaving unsightly scars; and the main object of this treatise is to show that however good this practice may be in surgery, it is exceedingly bad in medicine. Allopaths who know nothing of actual cure have some excuse for having recourse to operative measures; but it is the province of Homœopathy to show the world the true method of dealing with the diseased human organism, and I publish this treatise as a practical protest against surgical interference with diseased lymphatic glands. Surgery (apart from the surgery of accidents) is no cure; it only gives the semblance of cure by cutting away diseased structures, whilst leaving the seeds of disease behind. It is not infrequently a useful second best; but the thing to be aimed at in all cases is constitutional cure.

Gland diseases and Bone diseases are often very closely allied, and I have therefore included in the treatise a consideration of both, and also of the condition called Scrofula, on which both frequently depend.

JOHN H. CLARKE.

30 CLARGES STREET,
PICCADILLY, W.

CHAPTER I.

My First Lesson.

Case I.—Abscess in Armpit Dispersed without Operation.

IT is one of the canons of old school medicine that as soon as matter or pus has undoubtedly formed in an inflamed part, there is nothing for it but to let the matter out. There is no possibility, it is taught, of causing absorption of matter: when once formed an abscess must be opened. That impression is so firmly drilled into students in the ordinary schools,

A

that two years of homœopathic practice had failed to get it out of my mind. The preceptor who finally cured me of it was a very humble person—a hawker who came to consult me at the Homœopathic Dispensary in Ipswich, where I was then practising, for a swelling under her arm. On examining the part I found the whole armpit converted into a bag of pus. I said to her that it was an abscess, and would have to be opened, and I proceeded to make arrangements for the little operation. But I had reckoned without my patient. An operation of even that trifling nature she sturdily refused to agree to. I felt that the dignity of the whole profession was outraged in my person by this rejection of my advice, but I pocketed my pride for the time being and prescribed *Hepar sulph.* 6, one pilule three or four times a day. On her return the following week I expected to find that the abscess had opened itself in a very unscientific way, after causing much needless suffering to the patient. In this I was disappointed: she had gauged my therapeutical powers better than I had been able to do myself—the swelling was very much less! No opening had taken place, the patient was feeling much better, and the pus was nearly all absorbed. In a short time all fluid had gone, and an agglomerated mass of glands was left. The glands soon separated and then resumed their ordinary state, the patient recovering perfectly with a whole skin!

From that patient's "obstinacy," as I regarded it at the time, I learned a lesson which has been of the greatest service to me ever since. Matter *can* be absorbed, and its absorption *can* be promoted, by homœopathic medicines. When matter is absorbed in this way, it is dealt with as the organism deals with all waste tissues, and is not "dispersed" into the circulation to poison other parts. When matter can be thus dealt with, by putting the organism into a more wholesome condition, it is infinitely better for the patient to avoid any operative interference.

CHAPTER II.

Anatomy and Physiology of the Glands.

IN ordinary language a "gland" means a gland of the lymphatic system. It is in this sense that I use the term in the present treatise. Anatomically speaking, all the organs of the body which secrete definite fluids, such as the liver, the kidneys, the salivary glands, the sweat and sebaceous glands of the skin, and also some organs which have no known secretion, as the pineal and thyroid bodies, are glands. But when the word gland is used absolutely, it is the lymphatic glands which are understood to be meant.

The lymphatic glands are little bodies varying in size from a lentil to an almond, and are very widely distributed over the body. They are like so many "locks" on the system of lymph canals, which form a network of vessels spread over the whole of the soft tissues. The office of these vessels is to take up the used-up materials of the body, pass them on to the lymphatic glands, which so act on them as to make them again fit to be poured into the current of the blood.

In the ordinary course of events the glands are very well able to discharge their functions, but at times extra pressure is put upon them. When one has a gathered finger, instead of the ordinary amount of waste products of the part, there is a great increase, and some of them are of a highly irritating character. In consequence of this we often find a red streak running up the arm from the injured finger to the armpit, and in the armpit one or more enlarged and painful glands. This means that the irritating matters are being dealt with by the glands. These may prove equal to the strain put on them, or they may inflame and suppurate themselves.

On dissection the lymphatic glands are found to consist of a capsule, and an internal portion composed of pouches communicating with each other, and richly supplied with blood-vessels and nerves. The pouches contain "a molecular fluid in which numerous nuclei and a few cells may be found in all stages of development"—(Bennett). There are lymphatic vessels leading into the glands and others leading away from the glands. The lymphatic vessels are provided with valves which only permit the fluid they contain to travel in one direction, away from the surface in the direction of the heart. Those vessels which enter a gland open into the lymph spaces of the outer portion of the gland; those which leave it are connected with the internal portion.

The distribution of the glands is very extensive. The chief localities in which they are found are the neck, the armpits, and the groins externally, and internally under the lining membrane of the abdominal cavity (peritoneum), and in the folds of it, where it forms the band of attachment for the bowels (mesentery), and in the chest along the larger bronchial tubes, at the root of the lungs, and at the base of the heart.

It will easily be understood that the function of this system of glands and vessels is of very great importance. The apparently solid tissues of the body are in a constant state of flux, of building up and of decay, and on the regular discharge of this process of interchange (*metabolism*, the scientific call it) the health of the body depends. It is one function of the lymphatics to take up the waste materials of the tissues and re-organise them, so far as they are capable of it, for the rebuilding of the same or other tissues. If they act too sluggishly the tissues become thick and unhealthy, and a state of obesity, either local or general, may result; if they act too energetically the opposite condition of wasting will ensue.

But they have another function of enormous importance in the economy. I have spoken of the familiar instance of glands inflaming in the armpit when there is inflammation of some part of the arm or hand. The lymphatics, therefore, not only deal with the waste of the body, they attack the products of diseased action, and, so far as they can, destroy the virus of disease.

I will not rest content with my own authority on this point. The *Lancet* of May 12, 1894, reports a discussion on a paper by Dr Walter Carr, entitled "The Starting-points of Tubercular Disease in Children." In the report of the discussion which followed I find the following :—

"Dr Routh pointed out the value of the lymphatic glands *as a means of arresting the disease*, in the same way that the poison of syphilis or of a dissection wound was arrested."

"Dr Carr, in reply, said . . . he believed that the glands were usually infected near the primary source of infection. *He had no doubt that the lymphatic glands did act as filters and arrested the disease.*"

Closely allied with the lymphatics are the tonsils, which are looked upon by many surgeons as useless incumbrances (from the patient's point of view), liable to become enlarged from the slightest provocation, and good for nothing except for providing the surgeon with the work of cutting them out. But even in regard to the tonsils some authorities in the old school are waking up to the fact that they may have been put where they are for some useful purpose, and not solely for the surgeon's benefit. I quote the following from the *Homœopathic World* of April 1893 :—

The Tonsils.

In the *Revue Homœopathique Belge* of December 1892, Dr Martiny adduces weighty reasons against excising or even cauterising the tonsils. He quotes from a work (*Études Générales et Pratiques sur la Phthisie*) by Dr Pidoux, which was accorded by the Faculty of Medicine the prize of 10,000 fr. founded by Dr Lacaye, and in which facts were adduced to show that in phthisical patients the excision of the tonsils materially increased the predisposition to the disease. Says Pidoux :—

"I act in regard to the follicular angina of phthisis as with hypertrophied tonsils, which I never excise, no more than I do the uvula in phthisics or in those who appear to me threatened with becoming such; as also with anal fistula, skin affections, pains, leucorrhea, &c., &c."

And further on he says :—

"Now it is quite certain hypertrophy of the tonsils is one of the most benign and most natural expressions of non-degenerated struma (*des strumes non dégénérées*). It is often such with all the other characters of simple and nascent scrofula, in infants and strong adolescents, well formed, of healthy colour, with the aspect a little humid and full of juices. It must be feared, then, that the violent suppression of this primitive affection may be followed, in a predisposed subject, with pulmonary manifestations of catarrhal pus and still more retrogressive ultimates."

Dr Martiny adds that the above entirely agrees with his opinion. For a long time he has advised neither removal nor cauterisation of the tonsils; for he has discovered, on inquiring into the antecedents of consumptive patients, that a large number had formerly submitted to excision of the tonsils. For many years he has not met with a case of enlargement of tonsils that did not improve so much under treatment as to render their removal unnecessary.

Dr Martiny maintains that though nobody knows exactly what part the tonsils play as glands in the economy, this is no reason for concluding that they are useless; and that "to excise, to lacerate, to cauterise deeply an organ which exists normally in the human species and in a large number of animals," has always appeared to him the reverse of prudent.

CHAPTER III.

SURGICAL INTERFERENCE.

FROM what I have said above, the rashness of surgery in interfering with these vitally important organs when they are doing their office of destroyers and filterers of disease, will have became apparent to my readers. In the process of "arresting and filtering" disease, the glands sometimes become over-burdened, and inflammation and abscess takes place. But they are discharging their functions all the time. If they cannot arrest disease without becoming inflamed, the next best thing is for them to do it by suppuration. By homœopathic treatment, as my first case showed me, and as I shall prove by other cases later on, it is possible to so assist them in their operations as to prevent the necessity of suppuration, and even to enable them to remove the products of suppuration without opening externally; but even without homœopathic treatment it is far kinder to the patient to let the glands take their course and leave their own scars, than to cut them out and leave only the neat scar of the surgeon. How often do we not see in phthisical families that those who have on their necks the marks of old abscesses have lived and become strong, whilst others who have not had this disease-filtering and disease-arresting process have succumbed?

It is not always possible to trace the remote results of surgical interference. After the operation the patient is often temporarily relieved, and is to all appearance quite well; and when the disease comes back again it is in such a different form that its connection is easily overlooked. I think, however, in the two cases now to be narrated the connection is obvious.

CASE II.—TUBERCULAR MENINGITIS AND DEATH FOLLOWING REMOVAL OF STRUMOUS GLANDS OF THE NECK.

Ronald P., aged 4, was admitted

to the London Homœopathic Hospital on Feb. 10th, 1892, with the following history. Some time before (the exact date is not stated in the notes), he had had strumous glands removed from the neck by operation. Two days before admission he began to be fretful, crying for no apparent reason. In the afternoon of the same day he complained of irritation in the back, and a rash came out in the form of a group of pustules which quickly burst, being very irritable. The morning before admission he woke up and found he could not stand. This lasted some hours and was accompanied by complete loss of sensation. The power and sensation gradually returned, and he found he could stand but not walk well. On admission he had an unhealthy appearance, but was not wasted. There was an eczematous eruption on the left shoulder, running and irritable. There was no pain in the back and no curvature. There was much loss of power, and defective sensation in the legs. When he walked he trod on the outer sides of his feet, and kept the toes raised. The superficial reflexes were less than normal; the knee-jerk about normal. His temperature was 100°. Passed water in bed at times.

Under *Calcarea* he seemed to make some progress, but on Feb. 22nd sickness set in, and on the 24th there was commencing optic neuritis. After this there were fluctuations.

March 3rd.—Very drowsy; semi-comatose; screams out when moved; no sickness; bowels constipated; marked *tâche cérébrale;* keeps perfectly still; pupils dilated, react to light. From this time he gradually sank, and died on March 8th—Cheyne-Stokes respiration setting in before the end. From the beginning of this seizure on Feby. 8th, the boy, in my opinion, had not a chance. It is, of course, impossible to say that he would not have had this illness in any case, but my own belief is that he would not. If the neck glands had been left to do their work, unsightly though they may have been, they would in all probability have "filtered and arrested" the disease, which was undoubtedly tubercular. Possibly it would have taken them years to have done it; but as it was, they were taken ruthlessly away in the midst of their restorative work. No doubt the patient was very efficiently "cleaned up." The ugly sores were all removed, and he was made quite presentable once more. But he was not cured of his tubercle —surgery never can do that. It developed again, and this time attacked a part much more dangerous than the first, and the organism, being deprived of the eliminative powers of the removed glands, was unable to withstand the attack. The common notion about the danger of driving in a disease has a very substantial foundation in fact.

The next case is one of a different kind.

CASE III. — TUBERCULAR DISEASE OF NASAL BONES AND VALVULAR DISEASE OF THE HEART FOLLOWING REMOVAL OF GLANDS OF THE NECK.

At the beginning of the winter of 1893 I was consulted by a lady, Mrs W., 56, who gave me the following history. She came of a very tuberculous family. When very young she had sore eyes. She had all her life been liable to rheumatism of the limbs. In 1870 she began to suffer from lupus of the nose. This was treated surgically and "cured." The following year it recurred, and was again treated in the same way. Afterwards she had polypus, and this was removed. Volkmann treated her in 1872. Seven years later the nose began to fall in from disease of the bones, and she has been under treatment ever since.

In 1886, as the result of a cold, she had enlargement of the glands on the right side of the neck. A year after, these glands were removed and were pronounced tuberculous by the surgeon who performed the operation. For a time she felt much better, but then the nose became more troublesome, and in 1890 she had to undergo a very severe operation, bone having to be chiselled away to open a breathing passage. When she consulted me she was complaining of nervousness and irritability, with attacks of palpitation. She was less able to walk or bear fatigue than she had been formerly. When I came to examine the chest I found the cause of the trouble in disease of the aortic valve.

In this case the sequence and consequence of the events are, perhaps, not as clear as in the first; but, at any rate, there was a history of a surgical "cleaning up" of the outer structures, followed by an attack on deeper ones, and to my mind it is clear that if for the skin and gland affections the patient had been treated medically instead of surgically from the first, she would have been spared the attack on the bones of the nose and the last development of all, disease of the heart.

I am confirmed in my opinion by a discussion on the subject held at the meeting of the British Medical Association at Newcastle-on-Tyne in August 1893, and reported in the *British Medical Journal* of Nov. 25 of the same year. Mr Pridgin Teale of Leeds, on the suggestion of Dr Clifford Allbutt, first performed the operation of excising scrofulous glands in the year 1881. Their guiding principle in this operation was—"that, whereever septic material is contained in the system, we rest not until it is expelled and its burrows are laid open and disinfected." At the meeting above referred to, Mr Teale spoke, and among other points referred to the ultimate effect of the operation upon health. In 23 cases he made enquiries into the subsequent history of the patients. Twelve of these were in very good health; three were in "fair health," which means indifferent health; five failed to report; three had died. Now these deaths are remarkable. One died of tuberculosis of the lungs; one died suddenly of heart disease, and one died of abdominal cancer. This was thought by those present to be a very excellent balance-sheet. This only shows how very modest are the expectations of old-school surgeons and physicians. Most of the surgeons who spoke dwelt on the encouraging fact that they had lost no patient as a consequence of the operation. In addition to the three cases of death in Mr Teale's practice, Dr Ashley Cummins of Cork mentioned two cases in which extensive operations on the neck and axilla had been followed by acute consumption, and Mr Wm. Thomas of Birmingham quoted a case of removal of "a large glandular mass which necessitated the division of the sterno-mastoid muscle, and drawing up some glands from the thorax. The wound healed favourably, but the patient died fifteen months after from extension of the disease to the bronchial glands."

Mr T. Barlow of London, president of the meeting, summed up the belief of the speakers on the question of medicines as follows:—"Drugs were of use for improving the general nutrition, but had little demonstrable effect on masses of caseous material." However, he was not so enthusiastically in favour of operating as most of the speakers. "There was little doubt as to the right treatment of glands which were actually suppurating,"—the old fallacy of which my hawker patient cured me—"but there were many borderland cases of enlarged glands in which one hesitated about immediate surgery."

This madness for operating (*furor operativus*, as it is called) is by no means confined to the operation for removal of glands. An eminent French surgeon not long ago entered a protest against it. "We operate too much," he said, "and it would be a good thing if we listened more to the protestations of our patients. Quite recently three severe cases have occurred to myself in which I was convinced that nothing but an operation could do any good. The patients, however, insisted on being treated medically. I told them that it was sheer waste of time; but they remained firm, and were rewarded by *being perfectly cured without operation*."

It is notorious that many needless operations are performed on women. Dr Routh (*Medical Press*,

May 9, 1894) mentions an instance in point. An eminent operating surgeon paid a visit to one of his disciples, who "triumphantly brought out two dozen specimens, which he had removed from women, in bottles, which *in almost every instance were free from guile.*" That is to say, perfectly sound organs have been removed, on the supposition that they were diseased.

The poverty of the physicians' department is not a little to blame for this state of affairs. It is not at all uncommon to hear medical students say, "Oh! I shall go in for surgery, there is something to be done in that; in medicine nobody knows what he is doing—it is all conjecture." This is quite true of allopathic medicine; but the Faculty ought to take shame to itself that it is true. Medicine is the frontier line of defence; to abandon medicine for surgery is as bad as for a general to give up all his outlying strongholds without a blow, and give the enemy a free march on the capital. The object of the general (and of the medical man) is to keep the enemy away from the centre, and avert the risk of dismemberment, by all the means in his power. This, as I shall show, is what homœopathy can do in a very large proportion of cases.

But it is not always the operating surgeon who is to blame. Such is the effect of modern doctrines, that some patients actually demand an operation when there is no excuse for it. They have a kind of weakness for being operated upon (*furor operativus* in a passive sense). Some months ago quite a list of cases of the kind were recorded in one of the medical journals. A number of patients insisted on having operations performed, and they were successful in finding surgeons obliging enough to comply. One man was so convinced that he had a tumour in his stomach that nothing would satisfy him but that a surgeon should open him and see. This was done, and nothing abnormal was found. But even this did not satisfy him. He was sure the surgeon did not look properly, and insisted on having it done over again. One woman was insatiable: she had no less than seven unnecessary and unjustifiable operations performed on her.

CHAPTER IV.

Struma or Scrofula.

SCROFULA, or Struma as it is also called, is a constitutional state which manifests itself in peculiarly intractable inflammations, especially of the skin, eyes, eyelids, and glands, and in a tendency to tuberculosis of the lungs, abdomen, or membranes of the brain. The constitution is generally inherited, but it is remediable, either completely or to a very large extent. The underlying cause of it all is the presence of the psoric "miasm" as described by Hahnemann in his

"Chronic Diseases." Though not identical with "psora," scrofula forms a large section of the diseases described by Hahnemann as psoric. It is analogous to constitutional or inherited syphilis, and not unfrequently the two "miasms" are combined in the same person.

Scrofulous individuals are much more susceptible to morbid influences, and are thus more liable to take colds and inflammations than other people, and when they do become affected, they are longer in getting well. The processes of life are more sluggish, and as the lymphatics are intimately concerned with the process of repairing waste tissues, they naturally suffer more almost than any other part. It is for this reason that in the public mind the presence of enlarged glands in the neck has come to be regarded as the sign and proof of scrofula. And though there are many scrofulous persons who have no diseased glands, and many who have had gland abscesses who are not scrofulous, still the popular view may be accepted as in the main correct. Abscesses in the glands of the neck are a very common sequel of the ordinary fevers of childhood—scarlatina, measles, chicken-pox, and diphtheria.

In a perfectly healthy state lymphatic glands are not discoverable by either sight or feeling. When inflamed and enlarged they feel like "kernels" (a popular name for them) under the fingers; and if near the surface are more obvious to sight. Simple inflammation of a gland does not make that gland scrofulous. The truly scrofulous gland is a gland affected with tubercular taint; and by the time a gland is affected the constitution is also affected. Hence it follows that the only philosophical treatment is one which is directed to the constitution, and seeks to so change that for the better as to make it heal the gland itself.

Case IV.—Chronically Enlarged Gland in Neck Reduced by Medicine.

In May 1893, I was consulted by Miss D., aged 14, who had a gland in the neck under the right ear, about the size of a filbert, which had been troubling her for three years. She was tall (had grown much lately), stoop-shouldered (possibly due to short sight), pale and delicate-looking. She came of a very consumptive family.

May 31.—*Bacillin* 100 every eight days.

July 1.—Very much better. Gland smaller but not gone. *Calc. phos.* 30 thrice daily. *Bacil.* every eighth day.

July 28.—Better. *Repeat.*

Oct. 28.—Gland all but gone.

I have seen her brother repeatedly since, and hear she has kept quite well.

CASE V. — GLAND ABSCESS IN NECK. ABSORBED WITHOUT DISCHARGING.

Matt. B., aged 11, a very delicate boy, was under my care for enlarged glands in the summer of 1891. Under *Bacil.* 200 chiefly he got quite well.

In February last, after a blow on the side of the neck, one of the glands under the ear inflamed rapidly, and by the time that I saw him, a few days later, there was already suppuration present, the sensation of fluctuation being distinct. I forbade poulticing, and treated him constitutionally — *Bacillin*, *Hepar s.*, and *Psorinum* being the chief medicines given. Maturation went on, but at no time did the matter seem like pointing, and I refused to open the abscess. On the 12th of March he developed measles, for which I gave *Morbillin* 30. In a few days all fluid disappeared. The abscess dried up. I sent him away to the country, and he came back with no swelling of the neck to be seen, and only the remains of the gland to be felt.

CASE VI.—SUPPURATING GLAND AFTER DIPHTHERIA IN EMACIATED CHILD. SPONTANEOUS OPENING. INSIGNIFICANT SCAR.

Herbert B., aged 5, but not looking more than 2, extremely emaciated, without any power in his legs, which were no larger than a three months' baby's, was admitted to the hospital in the autumn of 1893.

He had lived in an underground room without sunlight and proper food. Under *Bacillin* 200 he made progress, gaining very slightly each week in weight. Under *Thyroidin* 3^x he gained $\frac{3}{4}$ lb. a week. Then an attack of diphtheria threw him back, but he recovered well under *Merc. cyan.*, but it left him with swollen glands on each side of the neck, and on the left side suppuration took place. He received *Hepar*, and afterwards *Silica*, and no external treatment. The abscess opened spontaneously with a very small opening, and healed rapidly, leaving a scar so small as to be hardly visible. The boy then gained weight again, and was sent for a change into the country.

CASE VII.—ENLARGED GLAND FOLLOWING INTERNAL THROAT AFFECTION, SIMULATING NEW GROWTH. THREATENED SUFFOCATION. SUPPURATION AVERTED BY TREATMENT. CURE WITHOUT OPERATION.

I was sent for late on the evening of Oct. 31st, 1893, to see a boy, T. W., aged 18 months. Eight days before, he had been taken ill with sore throat, which caused him to make a peculiar noise in breathing. The obstruction to breathing had gradually become worse, till he seemed in imminent danger of choking. Two days before I saw him he had come out in little red patches, which only lasted one morning. He had also complained of pain in his ear. The practitioner who attended him was so much alarmed by his condition that he proposed examining the condition of the throat under chloroform, and operating if necessary. This the parents objected to, and sought my advice.

I found the patient looking very ill, sitting up on his mother's lap, as he could not be laid down for fear of his choking. He had an enlarged gland, painful and tender, on the left side of the face under the ear. Saliva was running from his mouth, and a discharge from his nose. He was very peevish and irritable, and exceedingly difficult to examine. He had very little appetite, and there was great difficulty in swallowing. The bowels were regular. The urine was scanty, slightly alkaline, and contained a copious deposit of white urates. The chest sounds were clear. Temperature normal; pulse 120. It was hardly possible for him to sleep, as he immediately woke up choking.

I was unable to examine the state of the throat on account of the child's condition, but it was evident that the whole difficulty lay in some swollen or paralytic condition of the soft parts at the back of the nose. The difficulty was all in drawing in the breath; he could breathe out easily. As there was no fetor of the breath I excluded diphtheria. There was much working of the alæ nasi. He was constantly picking his lips and nose. The last symptom decided me to give *Arum triphyllum* in preference to many other more or less appropriate remedies. I gave it in the 30th every two hours. I took upon myself the responsibility of avoiding surgical measures.

Nov. 1.—The next morning I found he had had a very bad night, had coughed more, in choking fits, but had more rest in the morning. The gland was less swollen and less painful. He had not taken any more milk. More running from the nose. He still picks his lips; still making the same noise on breathing. I now gave *Bromine* 30 every two hours.

At 9.30 P.M., the same day, I found him no better; the nasal obstruction was rather worse. I gave now *Laches.* 30 every ten minutes.

Nov. 2.—Very bad night. Breathing very bad; cannot lie down at all. More gurgling in throat. Clammy forehead. Much discharge from nose. Has taken a little nourishment, and in spite of the bad night seems a little better when awake.

℞ *Hepar* 200 every half hour.

4.30.—A quarter of an hour before I saw him he vomited white phlegm, very sour. Is crying because he cannot go to sleep. Is more lively when awake. His cry is stronger. The *Hepar* seemed to relieve him very soon. The neck is much less swollen. He is very peevish.

Taking into account his constitutional symptoms, somewhat ricketty enlargement of wrists and ankles, backward state of dentition, head-sweat, which he had till he was five months old, and also the fact that his father had had a foot amputated for some disease of the ankle, I gave now one dose of *Bacillin* 200, without interrupting the *Hepar*.

Nov. 3.—In the evening he seemed brighter, and wanted food. Slept an hour and a half this morning. Is better; breathing better. The bowels have moved twice: the first motion like white jelly and blood, very offensive; the second, slight, dark and offensive. There is now very little running from the nose; just a little dribbling of saliva. The swelling is still diminishing. He cannot yet lie down, but sleeps with his head on his chest.

Nov. 6.—Has kept improving. To-day for the first time I was able to examine the throat. I found the soft palate depressed and bulged forward on the left side. Tongue white; nothing like false membrane seen. Repeat *Hepar.*

Nov. 7.—Poor night. Breathing difficult. Passed a very dark motion. Lump less large and less hard. Every now and then a croupy noise in throat. Is brighter, and takes a little food. He screams if laid on left side.

℞ *Calc. phos.* 30 every hour.

Nov. 9.—Yesterday vomited undigested food twice. Swelling is larger; has extended lower down. Does not make so much noise in breathing. Tongue and roof of mouth white. I gave one dose of *Bacil.* 200, and followed it with *Phytolac.* 30.

Nov. 14.—One hour after taking the *Bacil.* he seemed altogether different, and has been steadily progressing ever since. On the 10th an abscess which formed over the two upper incisors burst, and he has been better since. Has a cough, and is unable to lie down. The cough is in fits, coming on almost every hour. I found slight dulness and some moist sounds at base of right lung. There was a case of influenza in the house at the time, and I attributed this cough to that cause.

℞ *Sang. c.* 30 every hour.

Nov. 16.—Has been better. Not coughing so much. Breathing better. Mattery discharge from nose in night. Not eating so well.

Repeat *Sang.*, and one dose of *Bacil.*

Nov. 18.—The cough has been very bad; worse between 11 and 12 at night. Vomited phlegm. Wheezing and rattling in chest. Nostrils sore. Has a fit of coughing every quarter of an hour. Has difficulty with solid food. Glands much better. He is very cross.

℞ *Cina* 30 every hour.

Nov. 21.—Very much better. Brighter; appetite better. More discharge from nose. No longer picks nose or lips. *Right* side of the neck is a little swollen, but not at all sore. Still has a cough in fits, worse in the night or on lying down, but there is less rattling of phlegm in the chest.

Nov. 27.—Has got quite well in all general respects; runs about, eats and sleeps. Has no cough. Cold almost well, but he still talks thick. He lies on his face, and sometimes seems as if he would choke in his sleep. On looking into his throat I found still a large swelling at the back. The glands externally were insignificant in size. *He has cut three teeth during the illness.*

℞ *Bacil.* gl. iv.; *Calc. sul.* 3, 2 grains three times a day.

I saw him for the last time on Dec. 4th, when he was practically well. I gave another dose of *Bacil.*, and ordered *Calc. phos.*, leaving instructions with the parents to send for me in the event of his not getting perfectly well.

I will now give two other cases of a similar kind.

CASE VIII. — ENLARGED SUPPURATING GLAND ALLOWED TO OPEN SPONTANEOUSLY. INSIGNIFICANT SCAR.

K. G., 10, subject to enlarged glands and sore throat, had an acute attack of sore throat about the beginning of May 1892. He came of a rather scrofulous family, his elder brother having had painful abscesses in the glands, leaving scars. Two years before, he had had influenza. He had also had severe bleedings from the nose, and had never been quite well since. He was rather short of breath, and I found the mitral valve of the heart defective. When the acute attack was over, the gland, previously enlarged, became inflamed. Under *Bacillin*, *Silica*, and *Baryta carb.*, he made good progress, the cardiac bruit disappeared, and the inflammation of the gland limited itself. I did not allow any poulticing, but had it bathed with hot *Calendula* lotion. On June 30 it opened spontaneously by a very small opening, and healed without leaving a conspicuous scar.

CASE IX. — ENLARGED GLAND AFTER CHICKEN-POX. SUPPURATION IMMINENT, BUT AVERTED.

Robert M., aged 5, had chicken-pox in October 1893. There was a history of consumption on both sides of the family, and one of his father's sisters had suffered from enlarged and suppurating glands after chicken-pox. Whilst the eruption was out the boy had been exposed to a draught which played upon the left side, and on the same side a gland under the angle of the ear swelled to a considerable size and threatened to suppurate. A certain amount of softening took place, and any indiscretion in the way of poulticing would undoubtedly have precipitated that result. At one time during convalescence he caught influenza, which aggravated matters, but in the end, after persistent treatment, the gland disappeared without leaving any trace behind. *Bacil.* 200 and 30, *Calc. phos.* 30, *Arum triphyllum* 30, *Hippozænin* 30, *Arsen. sulph. rub.* 30, and *Calc. carb.* 30, were the principal remedies. The treatment lasted several months, but the result left the patient with a whole skin and an organism sufficiently strong to overcome the disease by its own efforts.

I will now give a few cases from what I may call the pre-Bacillin times.

CASE X.—POST-SCARLATINAL SCROFULOUS GLANDS OF THREE YEARS' DURATION.

Mary A., 9, of large growth, sanguine temperament, was brought to me at the London Homœopathic Hospital on the 19th of April 1881. For three years had suffered from enlarged and suppurating glands in the neck, which first began to appear after an attack of scarlatina. The father is strong, but has a depressed bridge of the nose; the mother is strong, and all the children are healthy except this one. Tongue rather white; appetite poor; cannot take milk; sleep good; is nervous; has had worms. *Calcarea* was first given, with improvement in general health; the suppurating gland had discharged.

May 28.—*Silic.* 6, pil. i. ter die.

June 16.—Complains that the pilules "made her sick and gave her diarrhœa." The neck, however, was much better; swelling much reduced.

Silic. 30, one pilule night and morning.

July 23. — Upper gland very much swollen; lower gland still discharging; general health good. *Repeat.*

Sept. 3.—Neck very much better; discharge ceased; health very much better. This was her last attendance.

Here is a case of less duration.

Case XI.—Enlarged Glands, with Eruption on the Skin.

Daniel W., 12, a thin, delicate, nervous subject, was brought to me on Feb. 25th, 1882, with enlarged cervical glands, and an eruption of sores on the back of the neck. The condition had lasted two months.

Bellad. 3, one drop in water three times a day.

Mar. 11.—Better. *Repeat.*

Mar. 25. — Better; once had some bad sores on back of neck, but now better; glands better.

He was now practically well.

Case XII.—Abscess of Neck and Inflamed Glands. Action of Aconite.

Annie D., 22, pale, nervous,

and low, came to the Hospital on Oct. 11th, 1884. She had had an abscess in the neck, which was opened at St Thomas's Hospital, where she had been for five weeks. Under the right jaw is an enlarged gland. Over the vessels of the neck there is heard the venous *bruit* indicative of anæmia.

Baryt. c. 6, one pilule three times a day.

Oct. 18.—Gland the same; has a very bad cold in the head.

Merc. sol. 6, one drop four times a day.

Nov. 15.—Has been absent, and for three weeks has had no medicine. Cold better; face about the same. *Repeat.*

Nov. 29.—Cold in the head is

better, but has a cough, worse during the day; raises much phlegm.

Mercurius s. 6, *Bryonia* 3, every alternate three hours.

Dec. 13.—Cough better; general health better; gland the same. *Repeat.*

Jan. 17, 1885.—Gland same.

Acon. 6, one pilule four times a day.

This completed the cure. Under *Aconite* the gland soon disappeared, and I quote this case in full to show the affinity of this drug for indurated glands.

CHAPTER V.

SOME CASES OF INVETERATE SCROFULA RESEMBLING "HODGKIN'S DISEASE," OR LYMPHADENOMA.

THERE is a disease of the lymphatic glands, called after the first accurate describer of it "Hodgkin's disease," which consists of an enlargement of the glands without much tendency to suppuration, but with much constitutional weakness, anæmia, enlargement of spleen, and an almost invariably fatal result. Though distinct in nature from scrofulous disease, the two affections are often so closely alike as to defy distinction, cases having occurred where the diagnosis was not even cleared up at the *post-mortem* examination. It is possible to have the two combined. The cases I am now about to relate were really, I believe, scrofulous in their nature, but they presented many points of resemblance to Hodgkin's disease. At the risk of being thought tedious, I shall give full-length pictures of these cases, as it is only by watching them over a course of years that a complete view of the disease in all its phases can be obtained.

CASE XIII. — DISFIGURING ENLARGEMENT OF GLANDS OF NECK WITH VERY LITTLE TENDENCY TO SUPPURATION. CONSECUTIVE INFLAMMATION OF THE EYES. FREQUENT COLDS. CONSTITUTIONAL CURE.

Charles M., 16, brassworker, consulted me at the Hospital on March 26th, 1884. For six years he had had very large glands on the left side of the neck and under the chin. Last winter, blotches appeared on his legs, and since then they come and go. Last winter, for the first time, he had a cough; it was bad for three weeks, and since then has continued to be troublesome. It continues during the day, and also in the night till he goes to sleep. He has a little swelling under the instep of each foot, which pains him when he walks. He looks pale. Family history negative.

℞ *Arsen.* 3, *Baryt. c.* 6, every two hours alternately.

April 16.—Feet and legs better. Swelling gone from feet. Cough gone. Has a contracting feeling in abdomen when he coughs; cannot get his breath for some time. *Repeat.*

May 7.—Breath better. Legs all right, but blotches have appeared on his face. The glands go smaller in hot weather, but this year there are more of them. *Repeat.*

June 7.—A gland under the chin has softened and discharged. A lotion of *Nitric ac.* 1^x, ʒi. to ℥vi. of water, was ordered, and healing took place rapidly.

July 2.—Great inflammation of conjunctiva. No photophobia; not much lachrymation. Matter; eyes red all round.

℞ *Euphras.* 1 every two hours; a lotion of φ tincture.

July 5.—Pain in eyes less.

℞ *Acon.* 1 every two hours. *Boracic acid* lotion.

July 19.—Eyes almost well. *Lumps in neck smaller. Repeat.*

Aug. 2.—Eyes well. Neck smaller. Repeat *Acon.*

Oct. 10.—Has a cold. Glands smaller. Have been still smaller, but have become a little bigger since the weather became colder. *Repeat.*

Nov. 12.—Neck smaller. Has another cold. *Repeat.* (Last year he had colds and coughs alternately.)

Dec. 10.—Cold soon got better. Glands smaller (they are usually worse in winter).

Dec. 24.—Has had another cold the last ten days. Nose very much stopped. Glands much smaller than they usually are at this time of the year.

℞ *Arsen.* 3 four times a day till the cold is better.

Jan 21, 1885.—Cold in nose still very bad. Glands smaller. To use *Vaseline.*

Feb. 4.—Eye has been inflamed. Nose less sore. Glands small. Has had sores on face.

℞ *Sacch. Lact.* *Vaseline* to nose.

Feb. 11.—Better. Nose getting better. Right eye sore still.

℞ *Acon.* 6 four times a day. Lotion of *Acid Borac.* for eye.

Feb. 21.—Eye a little better. There are two vesicles on upper margin of cornea. Nose better.

Mar. 5.—(Dr Moir, who was then in charge of the eye department of the hospital, kindly examined the patient's eyes for me, and prescribed *Puls.* 3^x, with the *Borac. acid* lotion.) Eyes better. Nose still very sore.

Repeat *Puls.*

Mar. 18.—Eyes much better, but still mattery. No pain. Glands same. Nose better.

℞ *Merc. sol.* 3, gr. ii. ter die. Lotion, *Borac. acid.*

April 1.—Nose much better.

April 15.—Better. Nose nearly

well, but a few days ago gland on right side of neck became very large. *Repeat.*

May 13.—One gland on right side has been larger, others smaller. Has a cough in morning on rising; dry. Eyes and nose keep right.

℞ *Bry.* 3 four times a day for a week, then *Acon.* 6.

June 3.—Cough gone. Face same. Two weeks ago had throbbing pains in feet and hands; now they are stiff.

℞ *Caulophyllum* 1ˣ four times a day.

June 17.—Feet and hands all right now. Has had eye bad for a few days; better now. Lumps about the same. A "pimple" came on the side of the eye as at first.

℞ *Acon.* 6 four times a day.

July 22.—Glands smaller. Two days after beginning the *Acon.* had a cold which lasted a week. Upper lip became sore and swelled. Nose does not feel sore at all now. Has pimples on face, chest, and back. *Repeat.*

Aug. 19.—Much better. Neck smaller. *Repeat.*

Jan. 6, 1886.—Glands smaller than ever. Has had cough three days. Gets up phlegm.

℞ *Calc. c.* 6, one pilule three times a day till cough is better, then *Acon.*

March 5.—Very much better. *Repeat.*

Jan. 12, 1887.—Lumps very small. Has a cough that seems to tear the throat. Slight cold.

℞ *Caust.* 5, one drop every three hours.

Feb. 18, 1888.—*Acon.* 6.

May 12.—Lumps rather bigger.

℞ *Kali mur.* 6^x, gr. ii. ter die.

Jan. 19, 1889.—Has kept well in meantime. Now has a lump appearing under ear. Repeat *Kali mur.*

Mar. 20.—Lump is larger. Has cough for a week.

℞ *Acon.* 6 ter die.

April 10.—Lump smaller. Has pain in feet and ankles; aching in limbs. Lumps of erythema nodosum, which feel bruised when touched. Eyes well.

℞ *Arnica* 30 ter die.

May 8.—Very much better. Soon improved. One or two small glands have re-appeared. *Repeat* if required.

July 13.—*Acon.* 6 ter die.

Sept. 15.—Lumps smaller than they have ever been. *Repeat.*

April 2, 1890.—Has had a cough three days. Chest sore. Irritability worse at night. Cough jars the head. Legs ache.

℞ *Sulph.* 30 four times a day.

April 16.—Cough gone. His chest is sore. Unable to lie on right side. Sleeps on left.

℞ *Psor.* 30 three times a day for a week.

April 30.—Better. Can lie on either side at night. Glands seem larger. Pain on left side when he laughs.

℞ *Acon.* 6.

May 16.—Pain gone. Slight stiffness in right arm.

Con. 30 ter die

May 28.—Feels well. *Repeat.*

I saw him for the last time on July 16th, 1890, when he was well, except for slight cold.

During the progress of this case, the great power of *Aconite* over the glandular enlargement was very strikingly manifested. It was the inflammation of the eyes which led me to prescribe it first, when the action on the glands was very marked.

CASE XIV.—CHRONICALLY ENLARGED AND SUPPURATING GLANDS. CONSTITUTIONAL CURE.

The case I am now about to narrate was under treatment upwards of three years. It presented some points of resemblance to lymphadenoma, or Hodgkin's disease. In this case suppuration had occurred again and again before the patient came to the hospital, and did so whilst he was under my treatment; but the gradual improvement in general health was most marked, and finally his constitution was able to get rid of the disease altogether. In this case, a radical "cleaning out" of the diseased glands by a surgeon would have necessitated the removal of almost all the glands the patient possessed,—and then the disease would have remained in the blood. The case exemplifies the necessity of steadily working at a case, though the progress may appear slow. The susceptibility to colds and coughs of patients suffering from diseased glands is worthy of remark. The glands bear the brunt of this vulnerability. If they are taken away, there is little wonder that vital organs are next attacked.

Fred. H., 26, polisher, consulted me at the L. H. Hospital on Nov. 22, 1884. He had been ill seven years with enlarged and suppurating glands in the neck and armpits, and he had also had abscesses over the breast bone.

He had, on admission, swollen glands on both sides of the neck, and one of them was discharging, having been opened ten months before. In the armpits enlarged glands could be felt. The spleen was rather large. The mitral valve of the heart was incompetent, but this was compensated, as the patient did not suffer from short breath. Tongue dirty at the back. Bowels rather relaxed; open, as a rule. There was no history of anything of the kind in the family.

Baryt. c. 3^x, one grain three times a day.

Dec. 6.—Neck more painful. *Repeat.*

Jan. 1, 1885.—Glands in neck have broken. Glands under arm have enlarged.

℞ *Acon.* 1, four times a day.

Jan. 3.—Still discharging. Abscess on sternum breaking out.

℞ *Calc. phos.* 3^x, two grains three times a day.

Feb. 28.—Gland on left side rather larger. One on right side discharges at times.

℞ *Calc. ars.* 3^x, one grain three times a day.

April 4.—Not so well. Glands more painful and larger. Scarcely any discharge. Gets faint at times. Bowels rather relaxed.

℞ *Acon.* 6, one drop four times a day.

June 6. — Glands larger and rather painful. General health pretty good.

℞ *Con.* ϕ, two pilules three times a day. *Con.* 30, one pilule at bedtime.

July 4.—Glands have been larger till the last few days. Now they have decreased. General health very good.

Sept. 12.—Has been at Yarmouth. There a gland broke, and discharged matter and blood. Other glands still very bad.

℞ *Acon. lyc.* 6, one pilule three times a day.

Oct. 10. — Lumps are bigger.

Have broken and been discharging. Since then easier. General health very good. Pulse rather frequent, but steady and strong. On listening over the heart I found the *bruit had disappeared.*

This showed that the competency of the mitral valve had been restored, and was a significant fact, taken in connection with the case of Mr Teale's, in which sudden death from heart disease followed operation, and the case of my own, in which disease of one of the heart valves developed after a tuberculous gland had been removed.

℞ *Kali iod.*, gr. iii. three times a day. A lotion of the same in the strength of a drachm to the ounce.

Dec. 24.—The patient remarked

to me, that before coming under my treatment he had always been better in winter than in summer. The glands have been larger in winter, but have broken out more in the summer. Since coming to me he has been better than before; no new places have appeared—only the breaking out again of old ones. *Repeat.*

Jan. 9, 1886.—℞ *Calc. Fluor.* 6^x, two grains three times a day.

May 8.—Feels much stronger. Glands same.

℞ *Acon.* 1, one pilule three times a day. *Acon.* 30 at bedtime.

Aug. 4.—No more abscesses. Lumps decreasing. General health very good. *Repeat.*

Nov. 27.—Has cold and cough.

Cough worse in morning with phlegm. Bowels confined for four days. Is stronger and stouter. Has a rather painful gland at the side of the larynx.

℞ *Nat. mur.* 30, one pilule three times a day.

Jan. 8, 1887.—Glands smaller; did not break. Cold got better. *Repeat.*

June 4.—Has had fresh cold and cough at night; cannot go to sleep for wheezing.

℞ *Arsen.* 3, one drop every three hours.

June 12.—Chest better, but still has cough on lying down at night. Aching all over. Has cold in head. Neck rather smaller.

℞ *Acon.* 1, one pilule three times a day. *Hyoscy.* 3, one pilule at bedtime if required.

June 24.—Cough soon left him. Still has cold in head. Aching gone.

℞ *Acon.* 1 three times a day. *Acon.* 30 at bedtime.

May 16.—℞ *Acon.* 6 three times a day.

Sept. 17.—Has been three weeks without medicine. Has had sharp attack of diarrhœa. Before this the right side of the neck swelled up much and then went down. It is both puffy and soft, but no distinct sign of pus. *Repeat.*

Nov. 12.—The glands did not break. Has had a bad cold and cough. Coughs much on lying down.

℞ *Rumex* 6, one drop every two hours.

Nov. 26.—Got rid of his cough in a week.

℞ *Baryt. c.* 30, three times a day. *Rumex* if required.

Jan. 4, 1888.—Has been well except for cold. Gland swelling again.

℞ *Acon.* 6, one pilule three times a day.

Jan. 28.—Very much better generally. The gland went down in three days. Cough less.

This was his last attendance, as he was practically well.

Case XV.—Enlarged Glands of Neck. Inveterate Case.

Alice M., 25, servant, came to the Homœopathic Hospital Feb. 11, 1889. She had had enlarged glands on both sides of the neck for

F

three years. The tonsils were not enlarged, and she could not account for their appearing. They were worse in cold weather and ached at times.

℞ *Acon.* 3, one drop four times a day.

Feb. 2.—Improving. *Repeat.*

Mar. 25.—There has been very cold weather. Up till then the neck was better. Not so well since. *Repeat.*

April 22.—Right side not so big, left a little bigger. Has had severe cold, but is better now. *Repeat.*

July 22.—Neck much smaller than it has been for a very long time. It always does get smaller in summer, but not so small as now. *Repeat.*

Sept. 2.—Better, but rather swollen since weather became so cold.

℞ *Acon. Lycoc.* 3, one drop three times a day.

Dec. 2.—Has been better. Now not quite so well. *Repeat.*

Jan. 6, 1886.—Glands have been painful.

℞ *Calc. Fluor.* 6^x, gr. ii. three times a day.

Feb. 3.—Better, less painful. *Repeat.*

Mar. 10.—Glands more painful in the cold weather.

℞ *Acon. Lycoc.* 3, gtt. ii. four times a day.

April 7.—Not so well.

Acon. nap. 1, one pilule four times a day.

June 9.—℞ *Kali mur.* 6^x, gr. ii. three times a day.

Oct. 27.—Kept improving under

same medicine till now. Has a very bad whitlow.

℞ *Silic.* 3, gr. ii. ter die.

The whitlow got better, and the *Kali mur.* was resumed. She continued under this for some months. On May 11th she developed a pain in the lower part of the back and right leg, which gave her much trouble. Under *Bryonia* it became much better, but did not leave her. Finally *Argent. nit.* 12 removed it, but she unfortunately had a fall, which brought it back again for a time. The neck steadily improved, and none of the glands suppurated, though at times there was a threatening of this. She ceased attending in December 1888.

CASE XVI.—INVETERATE CASE OF SCROFULOUS GLANDS. INFLAMMATION OF THE EYE. ACTION OF KOCH'S TUBERCULIN AND BACILLIN.

Ethel T., 12, school-girl, pale, sallow, very unhealthy looking, with enlarged glands on each side of the neck, and the marks of old scars, was brought to me on April 29, 1891.

Four years before had ophthalmia. The present swelling of the neck glands came on six weeks ago in consequence of a chill, as it was supposed. The right eye is inflamed, there being a phlyctenula at the edge of the cornea.

During this time her health has been worse. She has frontal headaches, a slight cough, is very irritable, low spirited, and cries.

Is chilly, and likes much clothing in the night. The tongue is white; bowels regular; the appetite is abnormally good, she is hungry before her proper meal-times. Sleep is bad; she wakes with pains in the neck and throat. She has large lips; they have been so for two years.

℞ *Acon.* 6, gtt. i. every three hours.

May 6.—Eye got very bad for some time; is much better the last three days. Much less pain in the glands. Is much better than she has been for many weeks. *Repeat.*

May 20.—Glands seem to be softening; no pain. The eye is bad. Many more phlyctenulæ have appeared. Eye feels hot.

℞ *Nit. ac.* 30, gtt. i. every three hours.

May 27.—Eye better to-day, but has been very bad. Glands inflamed and suppurating.

℞ *Hepar* 30, gtt. i. every three hours.

June 3.—Eye not so well for last few days; painful. Shooting pains in head.

℞ *Rhus t.* 12, gtt. i. every two hours. *Silic.* 30, one pilule every two hours if abscess opens.

June 10.—Abscess in neck opened spontaneously on 7th. Since then has been better. Has an itching eruption all round the body, and some spots on the arms. Had some of it three weeks ago.

Repeat *Silic.* *Calend.* ointment.

June 17.—Eye was better till last three days.

℞ *Sul.* 30, gtt. i. every four hours.

June 24.—Eye has been worse,

but now is better. Is low and weak. Feet hot; stockings damp.

June 27.—Eye worse; burning. Is low and weak. Worse in night; restless.

℞ *Merc. cor.* 3, gtt. i, every two hours. *Arsen.* 30, one pilule every two hours if required.

July 1.—Very much better; was better the next day after commencing *Merc. cor.* She can now bear the light and see a little. The rash is urticarious and leaves a scurf.

℞ *Merc. cor.* 6, gtt. i. every three hours. *Boracic acid* lotion (half a grain to the ounce). *Calendula* ointment.

July 8.—Eye better. Glands the same as before. Has had restless night.

℞ *Merc. cor.* 3.

July 15.—Very much better; can

see better. Has had neuralgia in teeth.

℞ *Conium* 30, one pilule three times a day.

July 22.—On 16th nose bled profusely. Pain in teeth has been bad; teeth carious. Neck better. Eye better, but there is still some photophobia.

℞ *Tuberculinum Kochii* 200, two globules on the tongue at once. *Kreas.* 30, one pilule every two hours if toothache continues.

July 29.—Toothache gone. Eye very much better. Neck better.

℞ *Sacch. Lact.*

Sept. 2.—Has been pretty well, but the eye does not get quite well. Ulcer in centre of cornea. Has had toothache.

℞ *Merc. cor.* 3, gtt. i. every two hours.

Boracic acid lotion. *Kreas.* 3, one pilule every two hours when toothache troublesome.

Sept. 9.—Eye much better; photophobia less. Has had much pain in lumps of neck.

Repeat. Also another dose of *Tuberc. Koch.* given.

Sept. 23.—Much better. Eye better; can write now. Toothache has been bad. *No medicine.*

Dec. 2.—Has remained fairly well the last ten weeks. All inflammation gone from eye. Leucoma on cornea.

℞ *T. Koch.* 200, three globules on the tongue.

Dec. 16.—Two days ago had pain in the side of the head and face, first on the right side, then on the left. The neck has been very painful; worse in the evenings; is now better.

Repeat the dose of *T. Koch.* 200. ℞ *Staphisagria* 30, every hour if required for toothache.

Jan. 6, 1892.—Neck very much better. *Repeat.*

Jan. 26.—Has been better. Neck better. Toothache at times.

℞ *Bacillinum* 1m., one dose. *Staph.* if required.

March 2.—Neck better. Has a very bad cold and cough; worse at night.

Repeat *Bacillinum* 1m. ℞ *Arsen.* 30, one pilule every three hours.

March 16.—Cough very much better. Neck better. *Repeat.*

March 30.—Has a suffocative feeling every evening. Glands

externally less swollen. *Medicine discontinued.*

April 13.—Face much better. One gland painful. Teeth better.

℞ *Bacillin* $^{1\text{ m.}}$ 3 globules.

July 29.—After three months, she reported herself as feeling better, but a gland under the chin on the left side is becoming larger.

℞ *Bacillin* 100, three globules.

Aug. 10.—Throat rather bad.

℞ *Bacillin* 30, three globules. *Calc. phos.* 30, two pilules three times a day.

Aug. 24.—Better. *Repeat.*

Sept. 28.—Abscess discharged inside mouth. *Repeat.*

In this case, one of the worst I have ever seen, the action of *Bacillin* had a marked effect in shortening the duration of the disease. The patient has recently reported herself for a slight relapse, but is much stronger than she used to be, has grown much, and in the interval has kept very well.

CHAPTER VI.

Non-Scrofulous Inflammation of Glands of the Armpit. Miscellaneous Cases.

I WILL now relate several cases of abscess in the armpit: the first, consequent on an injury to the finger; the others arising from constitutional causes. The three latter were connected with an eczematous condition of the skin of the armpit, the skin apparently often forming the starting point of the gland irritation. In each case a cure was effected by constitutional remedies, and without operative interference.

CASE XVII.—INFLAMED GLAND IN AXILLA FROM INJURED FINGER. SUPPURATION AVERTED.

Alfred T., 20, consulted me at the Homœopathic Hospital on Dec. 13, 1882, complaining of a swelling in the armpit, which he had had for a week. Two days before, he ran a nail into his hand; and about the same time he had a cold. There is a painful, tender lump in the armpit, about the size of a pigeon's egg. Appetite bad. Great restlessness.

Hepar s. 6, one drop every two hours. *Acon.* 3, one pilule at bedtime if restless.

Dec. 20.—All pain and tenderness gone. Swelling diminished. Hand also better. *Repeat.*

All danger of suppuration was now past, and the patient did not think it necessary to return.

CASE XVIII.—INFLAMED GLANDS IN BOTH AXILLÆ.

Miss T., 22, consulted me Oct. 24, 1892. She had been away in Scotland, which was her home, and had returned on Sept. 1st. She then had a swelling under the left arm. This was lanced by a medical man about the end of the month, and discharged a good deal. Now the lump had returned, and was painful and tender. She felt tired; had a sinking feeling from 10–11 A.M.; suffered from constipation with hæmorrhage at times; had cold feet, inclined to be damp; was drowsy and heavy in the day-time. Worse in damp weather; better in cold frosty weather. She received *Hepar* 6 four times a day, and the abscess soon opened spontaneously and rapidly healed. Afterwards boils appeared on the left arm. Under *Sulph.* 30, and afterwards *Nit. ac.* 30, she got quite well, and I did not see her again till the following February.

Feb. 3.—Has had a cold for a week, with influenza pains about her. During the same time had suffered from pains under her *right* arm, where I found two abscesses,—one the size of a bean, the other no larger than a pea. She had taken *Sulph.* on her own account. I now gave her *Hepar* 6.

March 22.—*Right* arm got quite well; but five days ago had a little pimple in *left* armpit, which broke. There is now a swollen gland, but

G

the pain is not in the gland, but in the site of the little pimple. There is not much itching in connexion with this; there was when the left axillary glands were inflamed before. I gave her *Rhus* 30, and she has had no trouble with her arm since.

CASE XIX.—INFLAMED GLANDS IN BOTH AXILLÆ FROM BLOOD-POISONING. SUPPURATION AVERTED. CONSTITUTIONAL CURE.

Miss P., 30, nurse, was nursing a case for me when she consulted me about herself, though previously she had been under allopathic treatment. This was on November 29, 1892. For two years she had had a succession of abscesses under the armpits—first under one, then under the other. They began whilst she was nursing a syphilitic case in hospital; but had been worse since she had had an attack of scarlet fever in the summer before I saw her. A sister of hers in hospital work also suffered from abscesses in the axilla. She suffered from headaches. Her hair falls out. She is worse at night. I gave her *Silica* 30.

As she was away nursing cases for long periods the attendance was very irregular. I did not see her till nearly four months afterwards.

March 8, 1893.—Has had five more abscesses, but got over them quickly. Hair does not fall out so much as it did. This was the first opportunity I had of examining the axillæ. Both were marked with scars ; the skin was red and eczematous ; the glands and lymphatic ducts were distinct enough to be felt. The pain was worse on exertion and at night.

℞ *Luesin* 200, four globules every ten days.

March 22.—Is more comfortable than she has been for months, in spite of rough work necessitated by nursing isolation cases. The glands have nearly all disappeared ; there is now no pain, but very great irritation in left armpit. *Repeat.*

This irritation has frequently been the precursor of an abscess, and proved to be so in the present case.

April 3.—An abscess the size of a small damson appeared in the axilla, and was so painful she had to poultice it for five nights to get rest. The pain has now gone; the lump remains, "but has ceased to press on something deep down in the armpit, as they all seem to do." The irritation under the arm is still troublesome. A small painful gland appeared in right groin. It was only painful two days, and was felt on walking. It has now gone.

℞ *Elaps.* 200, four powders. Each to be dissolved in a third of a tumbler of water; a teaspoonful four times a day.

April 24.—The patient wrote to me that for a day or two after beginning the medicine she felt sick. The sickness came on after the second dose. Such a thing never occurred to her before. The irritation under the arm was quickly relieved, and she felt really quite well.

May 13.—Patient called to see me. The armpits were irritable at times, and there had been one attempt at enlargement of axillary glands, and also of the gland in the groin.

℞ *Juglans Regia* 12, a tablet three times a day.

May 18.—Two or three days ago a rash appeared on the back, very irritable. It extended all up the middle of the back, from the sacrum to the mid-dorsal region, spreading out below and tapering above. There are minute vesicles. Aggravation by washing. *The armpits are much better;* very little irritation there.

℞ *Rhus. t.* 12 every two hours.

May 24.—Back very much better.

Armpits quite right. She is giddy when she takes a bath.

Repeat *Rhus.* ℞ *Coccul. ind.* 3, one pilule when required for the giddiness.

Aug. 28.—*Cocculus* relieved her of the giddiness. The armpits are quite well, except for a small circular eczematous patch, irritable in hot weather. Has a little glandular lump in left breast about the size of a large pea. She has been nursing a heavy case lately, and has had bad milk to drink. Has had violent headaches from vertex down over forehead and occiput.

℞ *Elaps.* 200 one dose. *Glon.* 30, one pilule every hour if required.

Nov. 27.—Writes to ask if she need "go on with any more medicine, as I am now so very well and strong. I can never say how grateful I am to you for having cured me."

I saw her again on March 22, 1894, when the arms were quite well, and the lump (which had terrified her greatly) had disappeared from the breast.

CASE XX.—INFLAMED GLANDS IN AXILLÆ ON SITE OF FORMER ABSCESSES. SUPPURATION AVERTED.

Mrs N., 35, consulted me in January 1893. At the age of 20, in Germany, had an abscess under one arm, which lasted six weeks. After the birth of eldest boy (aged 12) had blood-poisoning, and an abscess formed behind the left ear. In the autumn of 1892, had an abscess under the arm, which was opened, and continued for two months discharging and causing the patient a great amount of pain. The whole of the arm was red and inflamed. At the same time she suffered from inflammation of the bladder, which had left an irritability behind. For this and general debility I treated the patient at first.

March 11.—On this date I gave her *Sarsaparilla* 1m. four times a day. After this there was a sharp aggravation of the symptoms, followed by great improvement. Among the symptoms experienced was a sharp pain in an abscess scar in the left armpit. No more medicine was given.

March 17.—Has had no more

sensations under the left arm, but under the right has had pain for a few days. Now there is a little red spot visible in the skin. This is how the abscesses have begun before, and the patient is in great fear of a renewal of her old troubles. I told her I did not think the abscesses would come to anything, and if they did, I should not think of operating on them. On examining the armpit I found a little red patch of skin, and in the centre of it a gland which was tender.

℞ *Hepar* 30 every two hours.

Mar. 20.—On the night of the 18th there was throbbing in the armpit; on 19th there was soreness and inability to raise the arm. To-day there is less soreness. There is a good deal of irritation.

[The first attack of abscess began with itching in the armpit. In the right armpit there were five glands, which, however, did not suppurate. In the left there were seven, which merged into one large abscess.] *Repeat.*

℞ *Calend.* lotion.

March 23.—*Calendula* allayed the itching, but the glands are about the same.

℞ *Rhus.* 30, gtt. i. every two hours.

March 25.—Arm better. Less pain or irritation. Has a very bad streaming cold in the head, and diarrhœa.

℞ *Cepa.* 30 every hour. *Verat. alb.* 30, if required.

March 29.—There was great improvement in the arm, as well as in the other symptoms, but to-day the left axilla has begun to shew signs of activity.

℞ *Luesin* 200, one dose.

April 7.—Very much better; both arms better, but there is still a little irritation under them.

The dose was repeated on April 13, and afterwards *Hepar* 30 was given four times a day.

June 24.—The arms are more painful fourteen days before the monthly period. Still eczematous skin and little nodes.

℞ *Juglans Regia* 12, one drop with *Sacch. lact.* three times a day.

July 3.—Still a red spot in left axilla; all the time lumps have kept coming, but smaller and lasting a shorter time.

℞ *Luesin* 200, one dose, then *Calc. c.* 30 at bedtime.

July 12.—Has over-exerted herself and is not so well. There is a hard mass of inflamed tissue in left axilla, but less tender than it was.

℞ *Rhus t.* 30 every two hours.

July 15.—Much less tenderness. *Repeat.*

July 22.—A very red round patch, somewhat raised and rather moist.

℞ *Merc. sol.* 30 four times a day.

July 28.—Much itching on exposure to air.

℞ *Elaps.* 200, one dose.

Aug. 5.—℞ *Tellur.* 5 three times a day.

Sept. 6.—Arms well.

I will now relate two cases of acute inflammation of glands of the neck.

CASE XXI. — ACUTE INFLAMMATION OF GLANDS FOLLOWING WHOOPING-COUGH. ACTION OF *Lachesis*.

Herbert C., 3, fair, thin, was brought to me on Sept. 30, 1882, with acute inflammation of the glands on the right side of the neck, which had been noticed only three days. He had had whooping-cough, for which he was taken to Yarmouth. There had been no sore throat. The tongue was white, and the appetite bad. He complained of pain in the lumps, but he could swallow without difficulty and was not deaf. *Belladonna* 3 and

Baryta carb. 6 made some improvement, but not very marked.

Oct. 14.—*Lach.* 6, one pilule three times a day.

Oct. 21.—Gland very much better, much smaller, no tenderness at all. The medicine was repeated, and general health became markedly improved and the swelling disappeared.

Case XXII. — Acute Inflammation of Glands. *Baryta carb.*

Wm. M., 20, pale, sallow, anæmic, consulted me at the hospital on Nov. 8th, 1882. Four weeks before, he had a cold, and felt cold all over. After that he had pains round the loins, and noticed the swelling in the neck. No sore throat. General health good. Now has a large glandular swelling under the left jaw. It is painful at times, but not constantly.

Calc. iod. 3x three times a day.

Nov. 15. — Glandular mass smaller; glands separating. *Repeat.*

Nov. 29.—About the same.

Baryt. c. 6, one pilule four times a day for a week; to be followed by *Arum triphyllum* 1, one pilule four times a day for the following week.

Dec. 12.—Noticed much improvement during the first week; none during the second.

Repeat *Baryta c.* alone.

Jan. 3, 1883. — Lump almost gone.

I will conclude this part by

relating a case which I published originally in the *Homœopathic World* of Dec. 1, 1892. In this case the patient had already undergone an operation, and was on the eve of submitting to a second, when a few doses of a homœopathic remedy saved him all the suffering, and the surgeons their work.

CASE XXIII.—ABSCESS IN GROIN OF SEVEN MONTHS' DURATION. CURED IN A FORTNIGHT WITH *Silica*. OPERATION AVERTED.

On the 4th of July 1892, I was consulted by Mr ——, aged 31, holding a responsible position in a London house of business; naturally of excellent physique, but at the time looking anything but well or happy. He gave the following history :—Eighteen months before, he had had influenza badly. His eyes were affected, especially the right, and for a day or two he was blind. He became well enough to return to work, but his eyes had never got right, and he had never been anything like so well as he used to be formerly. Before the influenza he had never known what illness was.

In January of the same year, after a week of unusual physical exertion, though without any definite strain that he is aware of, he noticed in the left groin a little painless lump, which gradually increased. This he showed to his usual medical attendant, who painted it with iodine, gradually increasing the strength of the paint until the patient rebelled on account of the pain it gave him. This treatment continued for a month. As things were getting worse, he was persuaded to consult an eminent surgeon connected with one of the Metropolitan Medical Schools, who advised operation. Arrangements were made, and under ether the swelling was opened, the incision being made parallel with Poupart's ligament — for some inscrutable reason—and pus evacuated. This was in February. There followed a long, painful, and tedious convalescence. A gaping wound was left, and complete healing never took place up to the time I saw him.

Just prior to his coming to me

he had been in the hands of an allopathic medical man, who, after diligently probing the wound in various directions for three weeks, finally informed the patient that there was no chance of its healing until it had been laid open again under an anæsthetic. The patient's previous experience of an operation did not encourage him to face another; and before consenting, he resolved to try another system of treatment altogether, especially as he had been urged by friends to do so.

When he came to me, I found the following local condition. There were two linear scars in the left groin, parallel to Poupart's ligament, with several fistulous openings discharging slightly. I told him that in my opinion it would be a piece of cruelty to operate; that no good could be done by it, but that it would have the result of making an invalid of him and laying him aside for some time.

The fistulous openings in themselves presented tolerably clear indications for one medicine, *Silica.* The constitutional symptoms were meagre, but a tendency to moist feet, and a preference for hot weather, and sensitiveness to chills, supported this selection.

I told him to take reasonable care of himself, especially to avoid colds and anything like over-exertion, and to be careful about his diet. He was to use no lotion or antiseptic (or any application except what was required for cleanliness) to the wound, and as a medicine I ordered him one tablet of *Silica* 30 three times a day. He was to return and report himself to me in a month.

This he did. In fourteen days from the time he came to me all discharge had ceased. The wound had healed perfectly, and he was himself in better health than he had been any time since the attack of influenza the year before. In addition to this, his mind was relieved of the haunting nightmare of a second operation.

There still remained the eye trouble, which had lasted ever since the influenza attack. After ten minutes' reading he was obliged to desist from intense pain at the back of both eyes, with pain at the back of the head. For this I gave him *Conium* 30 and a lotion of *Ruta*. I have seen him recently, but not professionally, and he tells me that the eyes soon became quite well, and he has remained perfectly well in other respects ever since.

PART II.

DISEASES OF THE BONES.

NOT least among the baneful effects of specialism is the artificial separation of cases into medical and surgical. There is no use crying out against specialism: the enormous development of special departments renders specialism a necessity; but at any rate we may be on our guard against its dangers. There is no hard and fast line to be drawn between medical and surgical cases: most surgical cases are medical to start with. This is particularly true of cases of disease of bones. By common consent diseases of the bones are classed as surgical. This I maintain is a very grave error. In many cases diseases of the bones are perfectly amenable to medical treatment, and only when medicine fails should surgery be allowed to step in. Not long ago I dealt with this subject in an editorial article in the *Homœopathic World* (Mar. 1, 1894), entitled "Healing up" *versus* "Cure," from which I may quote the following passage :—

There is all the difference in the world between these two ideas,—curing a patient constitutionally and making a part heal up quickly. A true homœopathic cure of a patient leaves the patient for ever free from his disease; the removal of carious bone by operation, and the consequent healing up of the part, may take only a few weeks, but the "patient" is not by any means cured: he is for ever liable to a renewed outbreak. We have seen patients kept under treatment for years with frequently recurring bone abscesses; and by persistent homœopathic treatment the patient has been completely relieved of his tendency to the disorder, and has recovered with the perfect use of the limbs affected, and his constitution thoroughly renovated. This requires years of treatment, it is true; but it ends in cure and not in mere "healing up," which is the thing allopaths aim at. We are not saying that operation is never demanded: the circumstances in every case must decide: but the first thing to be considered is the *patient*, and not the diseased limb.

One reason why homœopathy makes no more progress in this country than it does, is the difficulty men have, in the present advanced state of the physical and, so to say, materialistic sciences, of apprehending Hahnemann's point of view. We constantly talk about "mind," "vitality," "the organism," but we are at great pains to explain whenever we do so that we really do not mean anything by the terms. "Mind" is the mere excretion of individual brain cells; "vitality," "the organism," are phrases to represent the sum total of the activities of all the cells of the body. Modern science has excluded the "soul" or the "vital force" from our confessed philosophic creed, although in our common speech it is perpetually cropping up. It was amusing to find in Dr Burdon Sanderson's Presidential Address at the 1893 meeting of the British Association the "living soul" re-asserting itself in that very centre of science under the name of "specific energy" which interfered with all calculations. "Heidenhain has proved," said Dr Sanderson, "that the process of lymphatic absorption, which before we regarded as dependent on purely mechanical causes, is in great measure due to the specific energy of cells, and that in various processes of secretion the principal part is not, as we were inclined not many years ago to believe, attributable to liquid diffusion, but to the same agency." Commenting on this passage, *The Times* had some very caustic remarks, reflecting on the philosophical acumen of physiologists in that it was possible for them so recently to hold such narrow and inadequate views of living things.

Hahnemann's clear vision saw in disease not merely an outward alteration of tissues and functions, but a disturbance of the living, "spirit-like" organism which animates the outward frame. This was to him the seat of all diseases (as distinguished from external injuries), and the remedies he employed were of the same "spirit-like" dynamic nature, capable of reaching the essence of the disorder. The cures wrought by Hahnemann's method are not mere "healings up," but realise the ideal of John Hunter: "What I call a cure is an alteration of the disposition and the effects of that disposition, and not the destruction of the cancerous parts." So long as so many homœopathists are *blinded* by the visible effects of disease, such as tumours and alterations of solid parts, to the alterations of the organic disposition underlying them, proficiency in the homœopathic art must necessarily be rare.

I will now proceed to give instances of the medical treatment of diseased bone, and will begin with a tolerably acute case.

CASE XXIV.—NECROSIS OF SMALL PORTION OF LOWER JAW: SEPARATION OF DEAD BONE WITHOUT OPERATION.

In my early homœopathic days, I was consulted by a lady suffering from an offensive discharge from the gum of the lower jaw. It was in a part where teeth had been extracted, and the probe showed the presence of dead bone. It occurred to me then that the best thing to do would be to take out the dead bone; but the patient was wiser than I, and would not consent. I therefore treated her with medicines—*Silica* and *Phos.*—and in a few weeks the bone came away of itself, and the patient was soon well.

This result was very much preferable to that of an operation, for many reasons:—(1.) An operation to remove carious bone necessitates the removal of a certain amount of healthy bone, whereas Nature makes a clean division between the living and the dead. (2.) The shock of an operation was avoided. (3.) The treatment of the patient improved her general health, and left her constitutionally better than before, whereas an operation leaves a patient constitutionally worse.

At the risk of being tedious I will give this case at considerable length, as it gives a good picture of the evolution of the disease, and shows how the disease of the bone was merely one symptom of a depraved constitutional state. Surgical removal of the dead bone would not have touched the constitutional condition, though it might have accelerated the healing of the sores.

CASE XXV.—SCROFULOUS DISEASE OF BONES OF FACE, HAND, AND BACK. PROLONGED MEDICAL TREATMENT. CONSTITUTIONAL CURE.

Frank C., 12, schoolboy, was brought to my clinic at the Hospital Nov. 22, 1884. Five years before, he began to suffer from scrofulous disease. Wherever he receives a blow ulceration takes place, and if a bone is struck the bone ulcerates. He has an open wound on the back, along which a probe passes for 2 inches, coming then upon dead bone (the sacrum). The face and right hand also affected. One of his brothers has rickets.

℞ *Silica* 3, gtt. ii. ter die.

Jan. 5, 1885.—Better; less discharge and less pain. General health better. Sometimes is ravenously hungry.

Jan. 24.—Has irritating pains at anus after stools.

Repeat *Silica*. *Teucr.* 1^x, three pilules at bedtime.

Feb. 14.—Irritation better. A

piece of bone the size of an almond has come out of the wound on the face. The back looks better.

Repeat. Add a lotion of *Silic.* 6 (ʒij.-℥viij.)

March 14.—Has passed many thread - worms. Now irritation gone. Has a cold.

℞ *Arsen.* 3 three times a day alternately with *Silic.*

April 11.—Has had hurt to thumb. Has a painful swelling under left malleolus. *Repeat.*

April 25.—Back better; face better. Thumb swelling has broken.

℞ *Calendula* ointment. *Silica* 3 and *Teucr.* 1x, as before.

May 23.—Has felt worse a little.

℞ *Cina* 1, three pilules at bedtime. *Silica* 3.

Aug. 29.—Side has healed up. Some pieces of bone have come out of thumb. Has cough; worst in morning.

℞ *Bry.* 3 every three hours. *Silic.* as before. *Calend.* ointment.

Sept. 12.—Cough better; better generally. *Repeat.*

Sept. 26.—℞ *Cod Liver Oil*, in addition to *Silica.*

Oct. 10.—A piece of bone has come away from thumb. Face healing. Back remains healed.

Jan. 23, 1886.—Another bit of bone came away from thumb. Often sees coloured lights, especially before right eye.

℞ *Calc. phos.* 3, gr. iii. ter die. *Calend.* ointment.

Feb. 13.—*Fer. phos.* 3, gr. ii., alternated with *Calc. phos.*

March 12, 1887.—Still improving. *Repeat.*

Sept. 5.—Hand much better. Pieces of bone have come out from time to time. Had a cold in June. Has had another, with sneezing and cough in morning.

℞ *Al. cep.* 6, one drop four times a day.

Sept. 22.—Cold still continues. Has been troubled with worms lately, and has passed many.

℞ *Teucr.* 1^x, one drop four times a day.

Dec. 13.—Cold persists. Worm symptoms no better.

℞ *Nat. m.* 6, one drop four times a day.

Jan. 14, 1888.—Cold not yet gone. Worms less troublesome. *Repeat.*

Feb. 18.—Throat nearly well. No worm symptoms. Has fresh cold.

℞ *Cepa* 12, one drop four times a day.

Mar. 17.—Gland in front of ear swelling, and behind neck. Still has cold.

℞ *Calc. c.* 30, one pilule three times a day.

April 28.—Fresh cold. Headache. Hand inflamed.

℞ *Merc. bin. c̄ kali iod.* 3^x, gtt. i. ter die.

May 12.—Cold better. Glands going down. Hand is better. Has bad taste in mouth.

June 16.—Cold better. Glands swollen about face. Still a little discharge from throat. Glands at times painful.

℞ *Sul.* 30 ter die for a week, then *Calc. c.* 30 ter die for three weeks.

July 21.—Has had toothache; bad taste in mouth. A new place has opened in the hand.

℞ *Iod.* 30 ter die.

Sept. 7.—Fresh cold. Glands bigger in face.

℞ *Hep. s.* 30 ter die.

Sept. 29.—Still has cold. Acne on shoulders.

℞ *Ac. nit.* 12 ter die.

Oct. 6.—Abscess in gland on face has broken. Thick white matter has come away. Cold better. Shoulders better.

℞ *Sacch. lact.*

Oct. 27.—Still has cold. Much defluxion from nose. Hand better. Face discharging and painful.

℞ *Silic.* 30, gtt. i. ter die for a week, then *Sacch. lact.*

Dec. 1.—Hand better. Cold in head again. Has not slept well lately.

℞ *Merc. b. c̄. kali iod.* 5 ter die.

Dec. 15.—Cold better. Hand better. Piece of bone coming out of face. *Repeat.*

Jan. 18, 1889.—Eyelashes falling out. Ringing in ears.

℞ *Staphis.* 12, gtt. i. ter die for fourteen days, then *Sacch. lact.*

Feb. 13.—Eyes well. Face better. Has another cold. Cough night and morning.

℞ *Ac. nit.* 12, gtt. i. ter die.

May 30.—Bad headache during the week. Ringing in ears at times. Hand better. Face bleeding.

℞ *Arn.* 30, gtt. i. ter die for fourteen days, then *Sacch. lact.*

July 6.—Bad taste in mouth.

℞ *Psor.* 30, gtt. i. ter die for seven days.

Nov. 7.—Varicocele of left testis. No pain. Has cold. Chills and heats. Bowels relaxed. Cough at 4 P.M.

℞ *Lyc.* 12, gtt. i. ter die.

Nov. 27.—Varicocele better.

℞ *Sacch. lact.*

Oct. 21.—Cough better. Still coughs from 4 to 5 P.M. Hand discharging. Repeat *Lyc.* 12 for seven days, then *Sacch. lact.*

Jan. 18, 1890.—Cough gone. Has had influenza. Hand still discharging.

℞ *Baptis.* 3, gtt. i. ter die.

I have recently seen this patient. He is now a well-grown man and in perfect health. His disease while it lasted was unsightly and tedious, but by the aid of medicinal treatment he was able to continue his avocations without being laid up a day.

I will now give two cases of disease of the bones of the spinal column: one in an infant, and one in an adult.

CASE XXVI.—COMMENCING POTT'S DISEASE OF THE SPINE. CURE BY MEDICINES ONLY.

Sydney W., the child of delicate parents, and born when his mother was far advanced in consumption, was noticed by his mother when he was fifteen weeks old to cry out when put in certain positions. On examining his back I found that the spine was distinctly more curved than normal, and one of the spines was prominent and tender to pressure. The boy had also difficulty in passing water and stools. When a few weeks old he had bronchitis.

On the 24th of July 1888, the day I discovered the condition of the back, I gave him *Calc. carb.* 6, four times a day. He was rather fat, of light complexion, and inclined to head sweat.

Aug. 20.—Still screams at stool and on passing water. Has a rash about him. Head sweat offensive.

℞ *Silic.* 6 ter die.

Aug. 31.—Bowels loose, motions slimy and green. Less pain on urinating. Has spots all over him. Looks pale.

℞ *Merc. sol.* four times a day.

He soon got over this attack.

Sept. 25.—Has many spots about him. Bowels confined. Cries before passing water.

℞ *Sul.* 200 three times a day for three days, then no medicine.

From this date he improved rapidly. The disease of the spine went no further. I treated him satisfactorily for various ailments, including a scrofulous condition of the eyelids, and he has grown a strong boy, with his spine perfectly restored.

In so young a child artificial supports were impracticable, and the medicinal treatment rendered them quite unnecessary.

The next case was one of a much more serious kind; but in this, again, medicine—that is, the specific medicine of Hahnemann—manifests its vast and inherent superiority to surgery.

CASE XXVII.—CARIES OF THE SPINE WITH PARALYTIC SYMPTOMS IN AN ADULT. ARREST OF DISEASE AND CONSOLIDATION OF THE SPINE UNDER MEDICINES ALONE IN THREE MONTHS.

On Jan. 15, 1889, I was consulted by Mrs P., aged 67. She lives in the country, but had come to stay with her sister in town to be under my care. She had had many illnesses throughout her life, but the present one dated from sixteen months back. In her village she was a very active philanthropic worker, and her present illness, crippling her as it did, was a great distress to her. She was fair, ruddy, naturally of a happy temperament. At present she was almost motionless from the pain in the back and chest occasioned by movement, and was very much shortened in stature.

As a child she was quite strong. At the age of 19–20 had "liver complaint" (intense cutting pain, vomiting of bright green stuff; was unable to lie down for six weeks). After this she had the "grape cure" in Germany. The following year had an eruption on her face. For this she had been given *Sulphur;* and had even had the sulphur waters of Cheltenham, but *Sulphur* always made her very ill. Erasmus Wilson treated her for the skin, and gave her *Strychnine* with benefit. She is still exceedingly sensitive to *Sulphur*, and cannot take it without its having a bad effect on the face. She had had bronchitis, jaundice, inflammation of the lungs, and years ago had abscesses, and on one occasion a boil. Has been married twenty-seven years. No family.

The particular points in the history of her present illness were as follows :—Thirty-five years previously she strained her back by lifting, and for several days was unable to do anything ; twenty years ago sprained her ankle. Five years ago had lumbago or sciatica. Fifteen months ago fell over some chains on a wharf, and had to twist herself in order to prevent herself falling into the water.

For a long time she has had pain up the back, nape, and head whenever she hurried. Sixteen months ago she noticed a little stiffness on moving in the morning. Then her head became drawn. She found great difficulty in turning round. Finally, her legs gave way, and she was unable to walk unless supported round the waist. Three weeks ago she became suddenly worse.

When I first saw the patient she was in bed, lying on the back, the head being unnaturally poked forward. She complained of pain under both scapulæ, the left being much the worse of the two. The pain seems to centre under the left breast, extending round to the left scapula and up to right shoulder. When she lies on the right side the pain is worse on the left, and *vice versâ*. The pain is constant, not periodic; it is relieved by lying in bed, and again at 12 noon, after getting up.

In the upper dorsal region is a large curve, caused by the giving way of several of the bodies of the spinal vertebræ. There was no tenderness on pressure.

Some months back the pain was constant in the right side below the breast, and at the back. She thought she must have cancer. Suddenly the pain went to the left side, where it remains. It was in

K

September 1888 that she first suspected there was anything wrong with the spine. The pain she described as like drawing the chest and back together; with sometimes jerking pain in cartilages of the free ribs. At times constriction all round, as if by a band. On account of the spinal curve the ribs are very much pressed together on both sides. When walking, she has a sensation as if she was walking sideways.

Among the general symptoms of the case, I noted the following:—She is rather deaf, but can hear well in an omnibus; in bed she is quite deaf. She is rather constipated; the water is scanty and high coloured. She perspires a little. For ten years she never perspired at all, when she was ordered a Turkish bath. She remained three hours in it without perspiring, but four days after perspired profusely. Feet dry and cold.

Here was evidently a case of rapidly progressing disease of the spine with accompanying paralytic symptoms. The indication was to arrest the decay of the bones and promote consolidation. There was no chance of restoring the bodies of the vertebræ which had collapsed, but if healthy action could be restored, new bone could be thrown out so as to form a kind of natural splint for the part. I was asked how long I thought it would take to bring about the change, and I said about three months. It was important to estimate the time, as the patient's sister, who undertook the care of her, could not continue it indefinitely. My estimate was fortunately correct. By the 15th of April the patient was able to walk up and down stairs unaided, and before the end of the month she was able to leave for her home.

There were many medicines which occurred to me, and especially *Phosph.*, *Sepia*, *Carbo veg.*, and *Lycopod.* *Phos.* has, in addition to its well-known relation to caries, "loss of power of limbs," and "tenderness of dorsal spine and muscles;" *Sepia*, "tensive pain in right side of back under scapula, especially when lying on right side;" "great aching between shoulders and under left scapula, extending into left lung, worse on expiration;" *Carbo veg.*, "stiffness of back, spine becomes bent;" "rheumatic drawing in back, worse on stooping;" "pain in scapular region;" *Lycopod.*, "burning in scapular region;" "drawing under scapulæ." *Lycop.* has also the transference of symptoms from right to left. I selected the first of these four.

℞ *Phos.* 30, gtt. i. *Sacch. lact.*, gr. ii., a powder every four hours.

Jan. 18.—Less pain in back and chest. Has had a return of some of the old lumbar pain, which has made her more helpless than she was. Bowels constipated. Since taking *Phos.* her mouth has become dry, and she has much thirst. *Omit medicine.*

Jan. 19.—Better; more strength; moves limbs more freely. Less dryness of mouth. Has profuse sweat of face; has had this for some months.

Jan. 21.—Stronger; less pain and stiffness. Throat less dry, but lips still dry—a very unusual thing with her. Bowels not yet moved; no feeling of it.

℞ *Op.* 3 every four hours.

Jan. 23.—Bowels moved twice. Much better generally; less pain in chest; no pain in loins; more strength in arms; can walk better. *Omit medicine.*

Jan. 25.—Has had a good deal

of pain on left side, worse at night, making her restless; nevertheless she moves more easily, and can stand better. She feels a grating sensation on one point in the back. Has very little pain in right side, but cannot lie on it. Bowels act naturally every morning.

℞ *Phos.* 30, one dose.

Jan. 28.—Had a very good night 26th, but not last night. Still has pain on left side, but moves more easily, can turn in bed, and can cross her legs when sitting. Throat is dry in the morning; roof of mouth sore. *No more medicine.*

Jan. 30.—Better. Less grating. Throat less dry.

Feb. 6.—Steady improvement till

now. There is tenderness to pressure over the spine of the most prominent vertebra of the curve, and she has a feeling as if lying on a bread-crumb when she lies on the back. She can sit upright in bed, propping herself with her hands. Holding anything in left hand makes her side ache.

℞ *Phos.* [1m.,] one dose.

Feb. 13.—Better. Can breathe better—almost naturally. If she sneezes she does not now have pain. Still feels pain left side on turning to right. *Repeat* one dose.

Feb. 23.—Has been making rapid progress, but now had slight cold and cough. Last spring had bronchitis badly. Has now more pain in side, throbbing at times and dragging down. A little flatulence causes a choking sensation.

℞ *Spig.* 1 ter die.

Feb. 26.—Better. *Repeat.*

March 1.—On attempting to sit up, all left side felt like a weight. Throbbing in side. No power to use arm except when lying down. Face flushed in afternoon. Roof of mouth and tip of tongue sore, but not dry.

℞ *Lycop.* ^1m.^ three times a day.

March 7.—Much better. Walks better. Pain nearly gone from side. *Omit medicine.*

March 11.—Back tender to lie on.

Repeat *Lyc.* three times a day.

March 18.—Pulse intermittent.

About fifteen minutes after taking medicine had heat at pit of stomach, followed by sinking. *Omit medicine.*

March 21.—Improving. Mouth dry.

℞ *Lyc.*, a few doses.

March 28.—Very much better.

April 4.—Not quite so well. Repeat *Lyc.*

April 8.—Legs very weak. Can hardly walk. Sinking sensation very troublesome. Constant uneasiness in stomach; very little appetite. Chest tight. Roaring in back of head. In spite of her sensitiveness to *Sulphur* I gave her a single dose of the 30th.

April 11.—Her side is better; she can sit up better, but is continually disturbed. Has hysterical attacks, bursting into tears; has a lump in the throat, and cannot breathe.

℞ *Ignat.* 1m.

April 15.—Better. Can walk up and down stairs. Can turn on right side and sleep on it. No nervousness. After *Ignatia* had the sinking sensation. *Omit medicine.*

April 22.—After a ride in a jolting bath-chair she was not so well. Loss of power in limbs, and weak all over.

℞ *Phos.* 1m. night and morning.

The next day was able to take a walk, and on the 30th was able to go to her home in the country. The loss of bone was repaired as far as it was possible. The curve of course remained, and the patient was much shortened in consequence, but she was able to return by degrees to her ordinary life, which was an active one, and included speaking in public.

A year afterwards I saw her, looking exceedingly well. There had been no return of the disease, though she had a little pain in the left side occasionally.

I will conclude with a case contributed by me to the last (third) edition of Dr Burnett's "New Cure of Consumption."

CASE XXVIII.—AFFECTION OF RIGHT KNEE. SUSPECTED INCIPIENT TUBERCULOSIS. CURE WITH BACILLINUM.

"A young lady of very good

physique, but coming of a scrofulous family (her mother's sister suffering from tuberculous ulceration of the nose, and her own elder sister having died after amputation of the thigh for scrofulous disease of the right knee), was taken last spring with pain in her right knee-joint. Being subject to rheumatic pains, she at first thought little of it; but as it persisted, I was asked to see her. Several remedies were given with but little success, and considering that her sister's illness had begun in a similar insidious way, her friends became somewhat anxious, and to some extent so did I.

"I gave her one dose of *Bacillin* 100, four globules on the tongue.

"Seeing her the next day, she asked me if I intended to make her knee very much worse? She said the dose 'went straight to the knee,'—at least within half an hour after taking it. She had violent pain in the joint, as after over-walking. This lasted for over four hours; then it went to the ankle on the same side, and then got better. From this time the knee began to mend, and in a few weeks was perfectly well. I gave other medicines afterwards, and did not repeat the *Bacillin* till a month after the first dose. This time it produced no aggravation, and was again followed by general improvement."

APPENDIX.

SINCE the foregoing was in type a paper on "Homœopathy in Bone and Joint Diseases," by Mr Gerard Smith, has appeared in the *Homœopathic Review* of August 1894. In this paper a case is recorded by Mr Smith which illustrates so pointedly my contention that the boundary line between surgery and medicine is in urgent need of reconsideration, that I cannot forbear to quote it in full. Mr Smith admits that the surgical treatment in the case was quite "correct" according to the recognised canons of practice; and yet, in his opinion (and, I may add, I quite agree with him), this perfectly "correct" treatment was the immediate cause of the boy's death. Could there be clearer evidence that the recognised canons of treatment need to be revised? I will now quote Mr Smith.

"I will mention one case which is instructive,—a boy of twelve, who, in November 1888, fell on the pavement while running, striking his right knee violently; acute synovitis followed. The joint, after complete rest for three weeks, *Aconite* and *Arnica* followed by *Bryonia*, apparently completely recovered soundness; but during the following month walking became painful, and the knee commenced again to swell without any rise of general temperature at first, but with the usual 'white swelling' and all the subsequent symptoms of a strumous knee-joint; the joint became very greatly swollen, and lost all the normal outlines, with the usual painful spots and general swelling round the joint; it was fixed in a poro-plastic support, the boy being confined to bed; *Silica* was given steadily, with occasional doses of *Bryonia*, for three months, when the joint had been reduced to nearly the normal size. Treatment of this kind was kept to for two more months, and the movements of the knee became again fairly free, though restricted. Active disease seemed at an end, and I had doubts as to the correctness of my diagnosis, since the knee scarcely seemed like one which had been affected with tuberculous disease. No doubt the joint membranes had not as yet become destroyed, and if there were any morbid deposits they were in the heads of the bones, and had presumably quieted down. A period of a month then passed,—the boy resting mostly on a sofa, and only walking with crutches, with the knee in a splint, and then, with no accident to account for it,

L

unless it may have been from cold, all the former symptoms came back, but with greater severity. The same treatment again prevailed to reduce the swelling and restore the movements; but a third onset induced the parents to take the boy to a general hospital, where the knee was excised, the articular ends of the femur and tibia being found full of caseous deposits, and commencing disintegration of the joint structure in evidence. After the operation all seemed going well, and the healing proceeded in a hopeful manner, but at the end of a fortnight the boy commenced to have some symptoms which were quite new to him,—he got severe headaches, which increased rapidly in severity, and were followed by convulsions. I need not go fully into the details: it will be sufficient to say, that after losing sight and hearing, and becoming entirely paralysed, the poor child died, and at the post-mortem examination there were found a cluster of tuberculous masses at the base of the brain and in the cerebellum, with widespread meningitis.

"I formed the opinion at the time that the operation had disturbed and set in movement the morbid deposits in the bones; this was a fatality quite out of the power of the most skilful surgeon to anticipate, and the operation was, by all rules of modern surgery, one quite justified; but I am confident that under homœopathic treatment the operation would have been much further delayed, and possibly a final recovery might have taken place without it.

"However mistaken I may be in this opinion, the case was one of great importance."

INDEX.

Acid borac., 67.
Aconitum, 60, 75, 79, 81, 83, 86, 95.
Aconitum lycoctonum, 76, 83.
Allbutt, Dr Clifford, first suggested excision of glands, 25.
Arnica, 70, 136.
Arsen., 64, 79, 131.
Arsen. sulph. rub., 55.
Arum triphyllum, 45, 112.

Bacillin, 38, 39, 41, 47, 49, 53, 55, 91, 157.
Baptis., 137.
Barlow, Mr T., opinion of, 28.
Baryt. c., 53, 59, 64, 75, 81, 111, 112.
Bellad., 58, 110.
Bennett on lymphatics, 8.
British Medical Journal, report of discussion, 25.

Bromine, 45.
Bryonia, 60, 68.

Calc. ars., 75.
Calc. carb., 55, 56, 69, 134, 139.
Calc. fluor., 78, 83.
Calc. iod., 112.
Calc. phos., 38, 48, 52, 55, 75, 92.
Calc. sul., 51.
Calend., 88, 107, 131.
Carr, Dr Walter, on starting-points of tubercular disease, 11.
Caulophyll., 68.
Caustic, 69.
Cepa, 107, 133.
Cina, 50, 133.
Coccul. ind., 103.
Con., 62, 76, 89, 119.
Cummins', Dr Ashley, cases, 27.

Elaps., 101, 109.
Euphras., 65.

Furor operativus, 29, 32.

Gland, definition and description, 5.
Glonoin, 30.

Hahnemann on dynamic nature of disease, 126.
Heart disease after gland removal, 22.
Hepar sulph., 3, 39, 46, 87, 93, 96, 97, 106.
Hippozænin, 55.
Hodgkin's disease, 61.
" " cases resembling, 63, 72.
Homœopathic World, extracts from, 13.
Hunter, John, on cure, 126.
Hyos., 79.

Ipswich Dispensary, case at, 2.

Juglans regia, 102.

Kali iod., 77.
Kali mur., 70, 83.
Koch's Tuberculin, 89.
Kreasote, 89.

Laches., 46, 111.

Lancet, discussion on starting-points of tubercular disease, 11.
Luesin, 100, 108.
Lyc., 137, 153.
Lymphadenoma, 61.

Martiny, Dr, on tonsils, 13.
Merc. bin. c̄ kali iod., 136.
Merc. cor., 88.
Merc. cyan., 41.
Merc. sol., 59, 67, 109, 140.
Morbillin, 40.

Nat. mur., 79, 133.
Nit. ac., 64, 86, 97.

Op., 150.

Phos., 128, 149.
Pidoux on tonsils, 13.
Psoric miasm, relation to scrofula, 34.
Psorinum, 39, 137.
Puls., 67.

Rhus t., 87, 98, 102, 109.
Routh, Dr, on function of lymphatics in arresting disease, 11.
Routh, Dr, on unnecessary operations, 30.
Rumex, 80.
Ruta, 119.

Sanderson, Dr Burdon, on "specific energy," 124.
Sang. can., 50.
Sarsaparilla, 105.
Scrofula, 34.
Silica, 41, 53, 57, 84, 99, 117, 128, 130, 139.
Smith, Mr Gerard, case of, 159.
Spig., 153.
Staphisagria, 91, 136.
Starting-points of tubercular disease, 11.
Struma, 34.
Sulph., 71, 87, 97, 147.

Teale, Mr Pridgin, first performed excision of the glands, 25.
Teale, Mr Pridgin, analysis of cases, 26.
Tellur., 109.

Teucr., 137.
Thomas', Mr Wm., case, 27.
Thyroidin, 41.
Times on Dr Sanderson, 125.
Tonsils, Martiny and Pidoux on, 13.
Tubercular meningitis after gland removal, 17.

Useless operations, Dr Routh on, 30.

Verat. alb., 107.

WORKS BY DR CLARKE.

Just published, cloth boards, price 1s.

HOMŒOPATHY:

All about it; or, The Principle of Cure.

THIS WORK CONTAINS—

"Sketch of Hahnemann's Career;" Chapters on "How I became a Homœopath," "Homœopathy and Allopathy," "Homœopathy and Pathology," "The Infinitesimal Dose," "Some Objections Answered," "The Hopefulness of Homœopathy," etc.

"In the following pages I hope to give a bird's-eye view, as it were, of what Hahnemann has done for the Art of Healing and for mankind. I have often been asked by friends and patients for some handy work on homœopathy which shall give them the means of answering their friends (medical and others) when the latter affect to put down homœopathy and its adherents with a few contemptuous expressions. '*We* know,' they have said, 'that the doctrine of Hahnemann is true, for we have experienced its beneficent effects in our own bodies, and *that* reason we can give, and it ought to be enough; but we should like to be able to do more than this, namely, to meet all the erroneous statements allopaths are constantly making about homœopathy.' Now there are numbers of works (especially the excellent publications of the Homœopathic League, from which I shall freely quote) which give the information needed, but not one which gives in handy form a sufficiently complete and compact survey of the question for everyday use. Such a work I have here endeavoured to provide. And I have kept in view (and hope to interest) not friends and foes of homœopathy alone, but also that large section of the community who have never found an opportunity of learning anything about the New System, either for or against. Finally, I have endeavoured to give a sufficiently comprehensive reply to those who have already advanced so far as to ask to be told 'ALL ABOUT IT.'"—*From the Author's Preface.*

RHEUMATISM AND SCIATICA.

Pp. 181. *Cloth,* 2*s.* 6*d.*

"This little book has apparently for its *raison d'être* the conveyance to despairing sufferers from rheumatism of the assurance that the answer to the question, 'Is there any cure for rheumatism?' depends on whose rheumatism it is; some people's rheumatism is curable, some people's rheumatism can only be alleviated, and there are some (a small minority, says the author) for whom no sort of treatment seems to be of much avail. That these prognostics are correct, Dr Clarke illustrates by the recital of the chief features of sundry cases of acute and chronic rheumatism, both simple and complicated with cardiac and other diseases, treated homœopathically. . . . . . The symptoms most resembling rheumatism produced in health by some twenty medicines are succinctly given."—*Homœopathic Review.*

WORKS BY DR CLARKE.

COLD-CATCHING, COLD-PREVENTING, COLD-CURING.

Third Edition, Revised. Cloth, 1s.

"A book for every house."—*Christian World.*

INDIGESTION: ITS CAUSES & CURE.

Fourth Edition, Revised and Enlarged. Cloth, 1*s.*

"These two little books, 'Cold-Catching' and 'Indigestion,' convey a considerable amount of useful common-sense information on colds and indigestion. The measures usually adopted to relieve the suffering each generally occasions are also sufficiently detailed, and the teaching illustrated by cases drawn from the author's practice. Both are written in an attractive and pleasing style, and they will, we doubt not, prove serviceable to those who follow the precepts they enjoin."—*Homœopathic Review.*

WORKS BY DR CLARKE.

CHOLERA, DIARRHŒA, & DYSENTERY:

Homœopathic Prevention and Cure.

Cloth, 1s.

"Cholera is a disease that needs treatment at the very onset, and if the treatment is not forthcoming the patient may die before a doctor can be procured. It is analogous in this respect to cases of drowning or rupture of varicose veins; anybody on the spot who has coolness and intelligence is bound to do what can be done without waiting for a doctor's arrival."

A BIRD'S-EYE VIEW OF

HAHNEMANN'S ORGANON.

Stiff Covers, 6*d*.

"A lecture originally delivered as part of a post-graduate series. It is from Dudgeon's translation, and is intended to serve as an introduction to a study of the original. It is an admirable condensation of this great work of Hahnemann, of which Dr Dudgeon thus condenses his estimate :—'Perfect and complete in itself, it leaves no point of doctrine unexplained, no technical detail untouched, no adverse argument unanswered.'"—*Medical Advance.*

"It will act as a worthy introduction to the Master, and make the study of the work an easier task."—*Minneapolis Homœopathic Magazine.*

"Treats succinctly of the main paragraphs of the *Organon.* Dr Clarke is a clear thinker and forcible writer, and his 'Bird's-Eye View of the Organon' makes many of the intricate problems of the book clear of comprehension."—*Medical Century.*

WORKS BY DR CLARKE.

THERAPEUTICS OF THE SERPENT POISONS.

Cloth, 1*s*.

"The book must be seen and read in order that its practical usefulness may be appreciated, the subject of 'Serpent Poisons' being treated most ably from a clinical standpoint."—*Minneapolis Homœopathic Magazine.*

"This little brochure contains an abbreviated symptomatology of *Lachesis*, *Crotalus*, *Naja*, *Vipera*, and *Cenchus contortrix*, from which much valuable information may be obtained. The characteristics and modalities are well and clearly given."—*Medical Advance.*

A DICTIONARY OF DOMESTIC MEDICINE.

Giving a Description of Diseases, Directions for their General Management and Homœopathic Treatment, with a Special Section on

DISEASES OF INFANTS

Cloth, 3*s*. 6*d*.

"Clear, concise, and reliable." — *Homœopathic Review.*